Physeo

TABLE OF CONTENTS

PEDIATRICS..8

Section 1: Child Development - Developmental Milestones & Growth..8
Section 2: Child Development - Puberty..12
Section 3: Glycogen Storage Diseases..16
Section 4: Lysosomal Storage Diseases Part 1...18
Section 5: Lysosomal Storage Diseases Part 2...20
Section 6: Inborn Errors of Metabolism..22
Section 7: Complications in the Newborn Period - APGAR Scores, and Extracranial Injuries........................25
Section 8: Complications in the Newborn Period - Neonatal Jaundice..27
Section 9: Complications in the Newborn Period - Respiratory Pathologies..30
Section 10: GI Disease - Hypertrophic Pyloric Stenosis, Intussusception & Malrotation with Volvulus...............32
Section 11: GI Disease - Meckel Diverticulum, Hirschsprung Disease & Necrotizing Enterocolitis.....................36
Section 12: Urology - Cryptorchidism, Vesicoureteral Reflux & Posterior Urethral Valves.........................40
Section 13: Urology - Penile Conditions...44
Section 14: Congenital B Cell Immunodeficiencies..46
Section 15: Congenital T Cell Immunodeficiencies - DiGeorge Syndrome...49
Section 16: Continental T-Cell Immunodeficiencies - Job Syndrome, IPEX Syndrome & Chronic Mucocutaneous Disease..........53
Section 17: Congenital Mixed Immunodeficiencies: Severe Combined Immunodeficiency & Wiskott Aldrich Syndrome.............57
Section 18: Congenital Mixed Immunodeficiencies - Hyper-IgM Syndrome & Ataxia-Telangiectasia.......................62
Section 19: Congenital Phagocyte Defects - Chronic Granulomatous Disease & Myeloperoxidase Deficiency..................65
Section 20: Congenital Phagocyte Defects - Leukocyte Adhesion Deficiency & Chediak-Higashi Syndrome...................68
Section 21: Congenital Complement Deficiencies...71
Section 22: Juvenile Idiopathic Arthritis...74
Section 23: Epiglottitis and Croup...79
Section 24: Bacterial Tracheitis, Pertussis, and Bronchiolitis...82
Section 25: Pneumonia..84
Section 26: Neonatal Sepsis and Meningitis...86
Section 27: Viral Exanthems...88
Section 28: Well-Child Care...91
Section 29: Well-Child Care - Physical Exam..94
Section 30: Child Abuse...99
Section 31: Acute Lymphoblastic Leukemia...102
Section 32: Neuroblastoma and Wilms Tumor...104
Section 33: Osteosarcoma and Ewing Sarcoma..106
Section 34: Neurological Diseases...108
Section 35: MSK Disorders - Hip Conditions..111
Section 36: MSK Disorders: Foot Deformities...116
Section 37: MSK Disorders: Orthopedic Injuries..118
Section 38: Bilious Vomiting...121

TABLES & FIGURES...124

We would like to extend a special thanks to the following individuals who have spent countless hours and support to make Physeo possible.

Ajay Davidson, MD

Alexandra Galel, MD

Alexandra Harding

Anissa Laine Bayabos Amilhamja

Anne-Sophie van Wingerden
Medical Student
Columbia Vagelos College of Physicians and Surgeons

Antonio Acevedo

Ayan Agarwal
MBBS Student
Vardhman Mahavir Medical College and Safdarjung Hospital
New Delhi, India

Brianna Cocuzzo, MsC

Brooke Walsh, MS

Camelita Thrift

Christopher A. Price, MS

Genevieve Saliuk
MD Candidate 2024
UTMB School of Medicine

George Myo Win, BS
University of Missouri-Columbia School of Medicine

Ghadeer Magdy Elshafey, MD

H. Robert Cannon, DO

Dr. Jabran Wasti, House Officer
Dr. Ruth K.M. Pfau Civil Hospital
Karachi, Pakistan

Jae Cheol Bae

Dr. James Nunn

Jennifer M. Locke, BA
MD Candidate

Justin Wong, DO

Kurestin Miller, BA
MD Candidate

Lauren S. Faber, MD

Lauren Schwartz

Lee Azolai

Leslie Jewett, MD

Logan B. Carlyle, OMS-II

Marisol Cárdenas Calderón, MD

Mark Parry, MD, Resident Physician
Department of Obstetrics and Gynecology
OhioHealth – Riverside Methodist
Columbus, Ohio

Mason T. Bennet

Mateo Betancourt Escobar
Universidad Autónoma de San Luis
Potosí, Mexico

Mohamed Elshennawy

Natalia Kerr, MD

Nijat Aliyev, MD

Nikoloz Karazanashvili

Nirupamaa Sivanushanthan
Medical Student

Ostapenko Karolina

Dr. Rahil Patel, Medical Officer
Sharda Hospital
New Delhi, India

Mr. Rishabh Goyal

Roaa Zayat, MD

Rojin Arefi, MD

Ryan Zia

Salikh Murtaliev, MD

Sarah Jaber, D.O.
Internal Medicine Physician

Sergio R. Ortiz, MD, MPH

Shawna-Kay Young
MD Student

Shelia Chandrahas

Soomal Zukhruf Memon

Sumit Raut

Syed Ali Haider

Syed Awais Ahmed, MD

Tori Walsh

Tamari Papidze

Telyn Peterson, OMS-III
Rocky Vista University
Southern Utah

Trey Edwards, DO

Warda Hameed, MD

Yasmeen Abdulrahman, MD

Yomna Dean, MS-4

Zurabi Zaalishvili, MD

PEDIATRICS

Pediatrics | Section 1: Child Development - Developmental Milestones & Growth

I. Developmental Milestones
  A. 2 months
    1. Gross motor: raises head and chest in prone position
    2. Fine motor: follows objects with the eyes past the midline
    3. Social/cognitive: parent recognition and social smile
    4. Language: coos
  B. 4 months
    1. Gross motor: maintains head straight and holds himself/herself on wrists in prone position
    2. Fine motor: holds rattle
    3. Social/cognitive: localizes sound
    4. Language: laughs
  C. 6 months
    1. Gross motor: rolls over back to front and sits unsupported
    2. Fine motor: transfers objects from one hand to another; raking grasp
    3. Social/cognitive: stranger anxiety; object permanence
    4. Language: babbles
  D. 9 months
    1. Gross motor: crawls and stands when supported
    2. Fine motor: pincer grasp
    3. Social/cognitive: separation anxiety
    4. Language: says "ma-ma" and "da-da"
  E. 12 months
    1. Gross motor: walks
    2. Fine motor: points to objects; 2-finger pincer grasp
    3. Social/cognitive: follows 1-step commands
    4. Language: knows 1-5 words
  F. 1.5 years
    1. Gross motor: starts running
    2. Fine motor: stacks approximately 4 blocks
    3. Social/cognitive: pretend play
    4. Language: knows 10-50 words
  G. 2 years
    1. Gross motor: jumps; kicks ball; walks on stairs with both feet on each step
    2. Fine motor: stacks approximately 6 blocks
    3. Social/cognitive: parallel play; rapprochement; follows 2-step commands
    4. Language: knows at least 50 words; speaks 2-word sentences
  H. 3 years
    1. Gross motor: walks on stairs with alternating feet; rides a tricycle
    2. Fine motor: stacks approximately 9 blocks; copies a circle
    3. Social/cognitive: gender identity
    4. Language: speech 75% intelligible; speaks 3-word sentences
  I. 4 years
    1. Gross motor: hops on one foot
    2. Fine motor: copies a square
    3. Social/cognitive: cooperative play; imaginary friends
    4. Language: tells stories; identifies colors
  J. 5 years
    1. Gross motor: walks backward
    2. Fine motor: copies a triangle; writes some letters
    3. Social/cognitive: dresses up; understands directions (left or right)
    4. Language: speaks 5-word sentences fluently

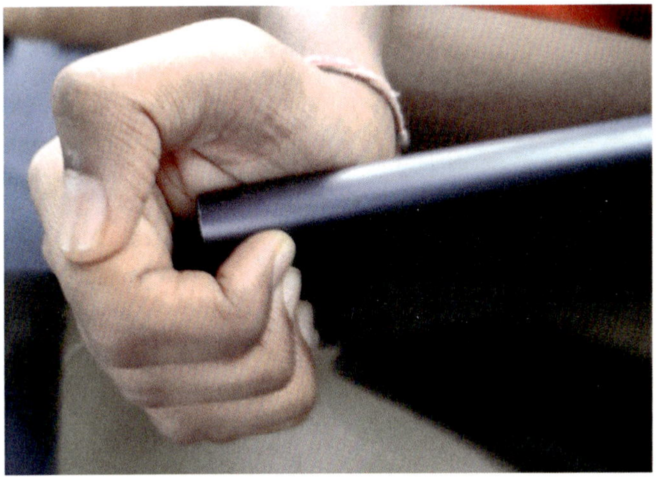

FIGURE 18.1.1 - Raking Grasp

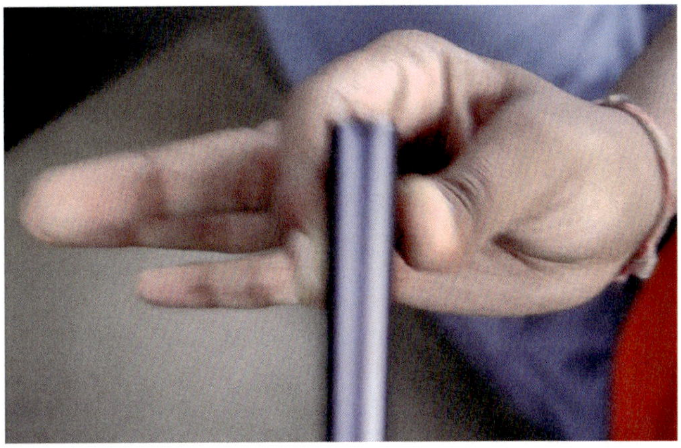

FIGURE 18.1.2 - Pincer Grasp

Age	Gross Motor	Fine Motor	Social/Cognitive	Language
2 months	- Raises head and chest in prone position	- Follows objects with eyes past midline	- Parent recognition and social smile	- Coos
4 months	- Maintains head straight and holds himself/herself on wrists in prone position	- Holds rattle	- Localizes sound	- Laughs
6 months	- Rolls over back to front and sits unsupported	-Transfers objects from one hand to another - Raking grasp	- Stranger anxiety - Object permanence	- Babbling
9 months	- Crawls - Stands when supported	- Pincer grasp	- Separation anxiety	-Says "ma-ma" and "da-da"
12 months	- Walks	- Points to objects - 2-finger pincer grasp	- Follows 1-step commands	- Knows 1-5 words

TABLE 18.1.1 - Developmental Milestones from 2 Months to 12 Months

Age	Gross Motor	Fine Motor	Social/Cognitive	Language
1.5 years	- Starts running	- Stacks approximately 4 blocks	- Pretend play	- Knows 10-50 words
2 years	- Jumps - Kicks ball - Walks upstairs with both feet on each step	- Stacks approximately 6 blocks	- Parallel play - Rapprochement - Follows 2-step commands	- Knows at least 50 words - Speaks 2-word sentences
3 years	- Walks on stairs with alternating feet - Rides a tricycle	- Stacks approximately 9 blocks - Copies a circle	- Gender identity	- Speech 75% intelligible - Speaks 3-word sentences
4 years	- Hops on one foot	- Copies a square	- Cooperative play - Imaginary friends	- Tells stories - Identifies colors
5 years	- Walks backward	- Copies a triangle - Writes some letters	- Dresses up - Understands directions (left or right)	- Speaks 5-word sentences fluently

TABLE 18.1.2 - Developmental Milestones from 1.5 Years to 5 Years

II. Growth
   A. Growth is tracked via growth charts depicting a child's weight, height/length, and head circumference compared to age
   B. Weight, height, and head circumference expressed as percentiles
   C. Normal weight-for-age velocity
      1. Neonates normally lose ≤ 7% of birth weight, and regain it within the first two weeks
   D. Birth weight
      1. Doubles by 4 months
      2. Triples by 1 year
      3. Quadruples by 2 years
   E. Normal height/length-for-age velocity
      1. From birth to 6 months: increases by 2.5 cm per month
      2. From 6 months to 12 months: increases by 1.3 cm per month
   F. Normal head circumference-for-age velocity
   G. Head circumference increases by approximately
      1. 5 cm within the first 3 months
      2. 4 cm from 3 to 6 months
      3. 2 cm from 6 to 9 months
      4. 1 cm from 9 to 12 months
   H. Failure to thrive (FTT)
      1. Length-for-age < 5th percentile
      2. Weight-for-age < 5th percentile
      3. BMI-for-age < 5th percentile
   I. Causes
      1. Non-organic (most common)
      2. Organic
   J. Non-organic causes
      1. Poor socioeconomic status
      2. Child neglect
      3. Inadequate preparation of formula
      4. Inadequate feeding
   K. Organic causes
      1. Cleft lip/palate
      2. Celiac disease
      3. Inflammatory bowel disease
      4. Cystic fibrosis
      5. Hypertrophic pyloric stenosis
      6. Gastroesophageal reflux disease

L. Diagnosis
M. Mostly clinical by investigating feeding habits
N. Laboratory or imaging studies based on suspected organic causes
    1. Treatment
O. Nutritional rehabilitation and parental education about adequate feeding
P. Disease-specific management for organic causes

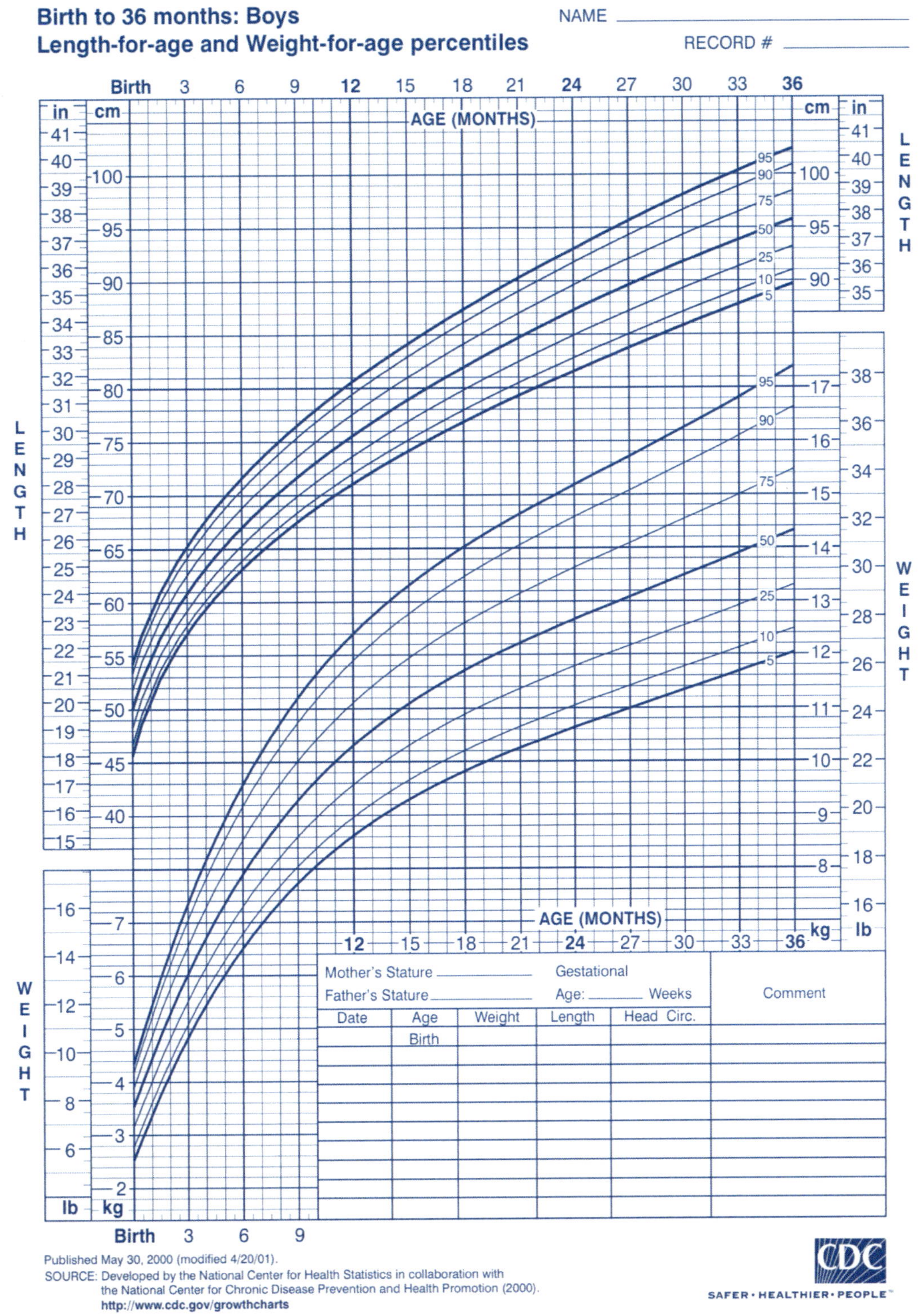

CDC, Public domain, via Wikimedia Commons

FIGURE 18.1.3 - Growth Chart

REVIEW QUESTIONS

1. A 4-year-old boy is brought to his primary care physician by his mother, reporting strange behavior for the last 6 months. The mother has noticed that the boy talks to himself in his bedroom when there is no one there. He is an active, playful child. He attends kindergarten and has several friends there. When the physician asks about his friends, he says, "my best friend is Mike. He is always with me, but nobody seems to notice him other than me." The mother asks if her son needs medication. What is the next best step in the management of this patient?

   - **The next best step in managing this patient is to reassure the mother about the normal nature of his son's behavior.**
   - This patient is an active, playful child with several friends in kindergarten.
   - This indicates that he is functioning normally in society.
   - His best friend is Mike, but according to the patient, nobody seems to notice Mike.
   - Mike is most likely to be his imaginary friend to whom he talks when he is alone in the bedroom.
   - Having an imaginary friend is part of normal development for a 4-year-old child, and it helps the child acquire social skills by practicing various social situations.

2. A 5-day-old girl is brought to her primary care physician by her mother for a routine examination. She was born via spontaneous vaginal delivery. Birth weight was 7.9 lbs (3,600 g)(2,500-4,000 g), and the length was 19.7 inches (50 cm) (48-53 cm). Vital signs include a temperature of 96.80 °F (36.0 °C), blood pressure of 75/50 mmHg, heart rate of 120 beats/min, and respiratory rate of 50 breaths/min. The mother says her daughter looks a little "skinnier than normal." The current weight of the baby is 7.5 lbs (3,420 g). What is the best next step in the management of this patient?

   - **The best next step in the management is to reassure the mother and counsel her on continuing breastfeeding.**
   - This 5-day-old patient presents with a slight weight loss.
   - Her birth weight was 7 lbs 9 oz (3,600 g), while her current weight is 7.5 lbs (3,420 g).
   - She lost .4 lbs (180 g), 5% of her birth weight.
   - Neonates lose up to 7% of their birth weight within the first five days and regain it within the first two weeks.

3. A 2-year-old boy is brought to his primary care physician by his mother for a routine examination. He was born at 39 weeks of gestation via spontaneous vaginal delivery. His age-appropriate vaccinations are up to date. He walks by, holding onto the furniture. He is able to stack 3 blocks on top of each other. The physician observes that the boy moves away from his mother and returns to her. He comes to the table and picks up a toy after being told by his mother to do so. Vital signs and the physical exam are unremarkable. Which of the following is the most accurate interpretation of this patient's development?

   A. Delayed gross motor, intact fine motor, intact social development
   B. Intact gross motor, delayed fine motor, intact social development
   C. Delayed gross motor, delayed fine motor, intact social development
   D. Intact gross motor, intact fine motor, delayed social development

   - **The correct answer is C.**
   - This patient walks by holding on to the furniture.
   - Normally, a 2-year-old child should be able to jump, walk freely, and walk on the stairs with both feet on each step.
   - Therefore, this patient's gross motor development is delayed.
   - He stacks only 3 blocks on top of each other.
   - Normally, a 2-year-old child is able to stack approximately 6 blocks.
   - This discrepancy between the normal and the observed findings suggests delayed fine motor development.
   - Finally, the patient moves away from his mother and returns to her.
   - He also follows a 2-step command by his mother.
   - This indicates intact social and cognitive development.
   - Option A is incorrect because although this patient has delayed gross motor development, his fine motor development is also delayed rather than intact.
   - Option B is incorrect because this patient's gross motor development is delayed rather than intact.
   - Finally, option D is incorrect because both gross motor and fine motor development are delayed in this patient while social development is intact.

Pediatrics | Section 2: Child Development - Puberty

I. Puberty
   A. Onset in girls: 8 - 13 years
   B. Onset in boys: 9 - 14 years
   C. Adrenarche: initiation of adrenal androgen production
   D. Gonadarche: initiation of gonadal hormone production
   E. Thelarche: onset of breast development; menarche: onset of menses
   F. Pubarche: onset of pubic hair development
   G. Sequence of changes in girls: adrenarche → gonadarche → thelarche → growth spurt → pubarche → menarche
   H. Sequence of changes in boys: adrenarche → gonadarche → pubarche → growth spurt → androgenic hair growth
   I. First visible sign of puberty
      1. Girls: breast development
      2. Boys: testicular enlargement
   J. Tanner stages (sexual maturity rating scale)
      1. 5 stages
         a) Depicts independent development of breast, genitalia, and pubic hair
         b) Three criteria assessed independently of each other (e.g. Tanner stage 1 pubic hair and Tanner stage 3 genitalia)
   K. Precocious puberty: development of secondary sex characteristics before age 8 in girls and age 9 in boys
   L. Types
      1. Central (gonadotropin-dependent)
      2. Peripheral (gonadotropin-independent)
      3. Benign pubertal variants
      4. Obesity-related precocious sexual development

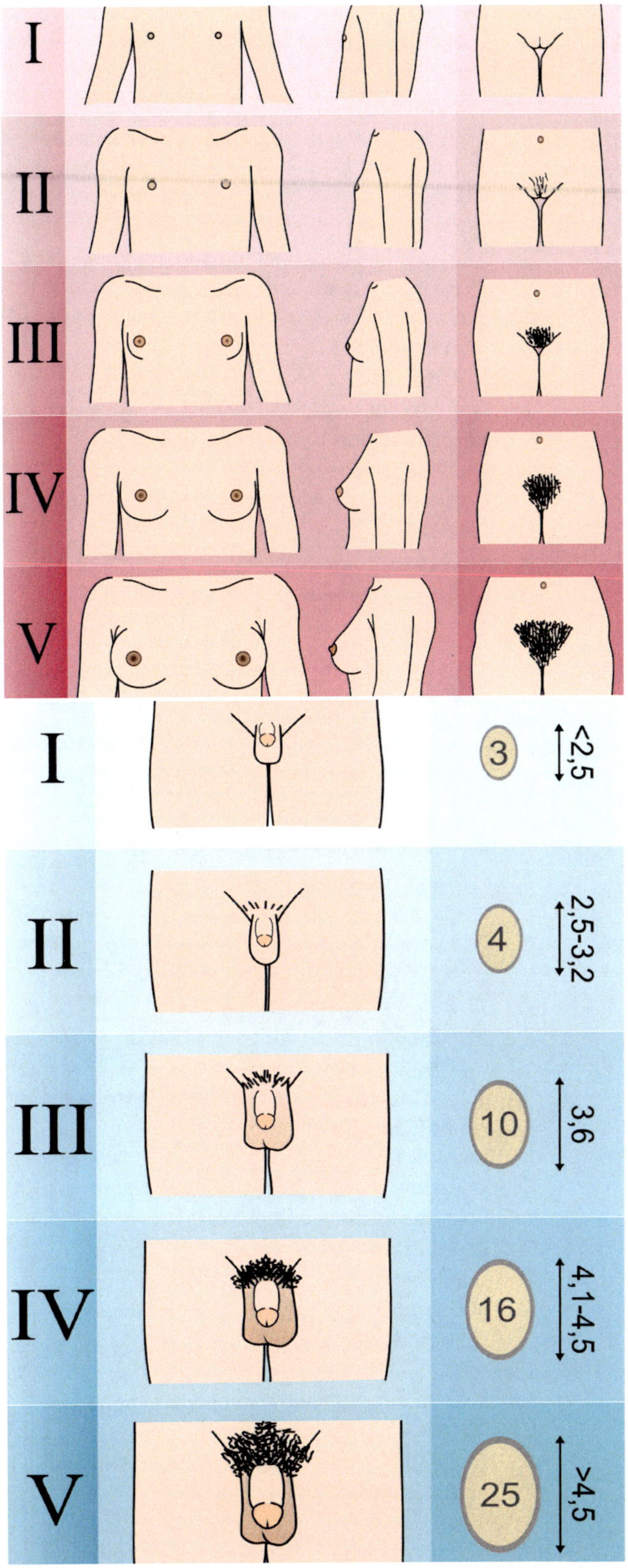

FIGURE 18.1.4 - Tanner Stages

II. Central Precocious Puberty
  A. Precocious puberty with high GnRH levels
  B. Causes
    1. Idiopathic (most common)
    2. CNS tumor
  C. Pathophysiology
    1. Early activation of hypothalamic-hypophyseal-gonadal axis: high GnRH, FSH/LH, testosterone, estrogen
  D. Diagnosis
    1. X-ray of hand and wrist to estimate bone age
    2. FSH/LH, estradiol, and testosterone
    3. Increased baseline LH or increased LH on GnRH stimulation test
  E. Treatment
    1. GnRH agonists (e.g. leuprolide) to prevent premature closure of growth plates
  F. Peripheral Precocious Puberty
    1. Precocious puberty with low or normal GnRH levels
    2. Causes:
      a) Increased peripheral sex hormone production
        (1) Congenital adrenal hyperplasia, ovarian cyst, Sertoli-Leydig cell tumor, McCune-Albright syndrome
        (2) Dysgerminoma and seminoma → hCG
      b) Exposure to exogenous sex hormones: androgen or estrogen
  G. Congenital adrenal hyperplasia
    1. 21-hydroxylase deficiency: hyperandrogenism with hypotension and hyperkalemia
    2. 11-beta-hydroxylase deficiency: hyperandrogenism with hypertension and hypokalemia
  H. Ovarian cyst (estrogen production) or Sertoli-Leydig cell tumor (testosterone production)
  I. McCune-Albright syndrome
    1. Unilateral sharply contoured cafe-au-lait spots
    2. Polyostotic fibrous dysplasia
    3. Peripheral precocious puberty
  J. Ovarian dysgerminoma or testicular seminoma
    1. hCG production - activation of LH receptors - increased androgen production
  K. Diagnosis
    1. X-ray of hand and wrist to estimate bone age
    2. FSH/LH, estradiol, and testosterone
    3. GnRH stimulation test (no change in LH levels)
    4. Abdominopelvic imaging
  L. Treatment
    1. Disease-specific: removal of tumor; cortisol in CAH

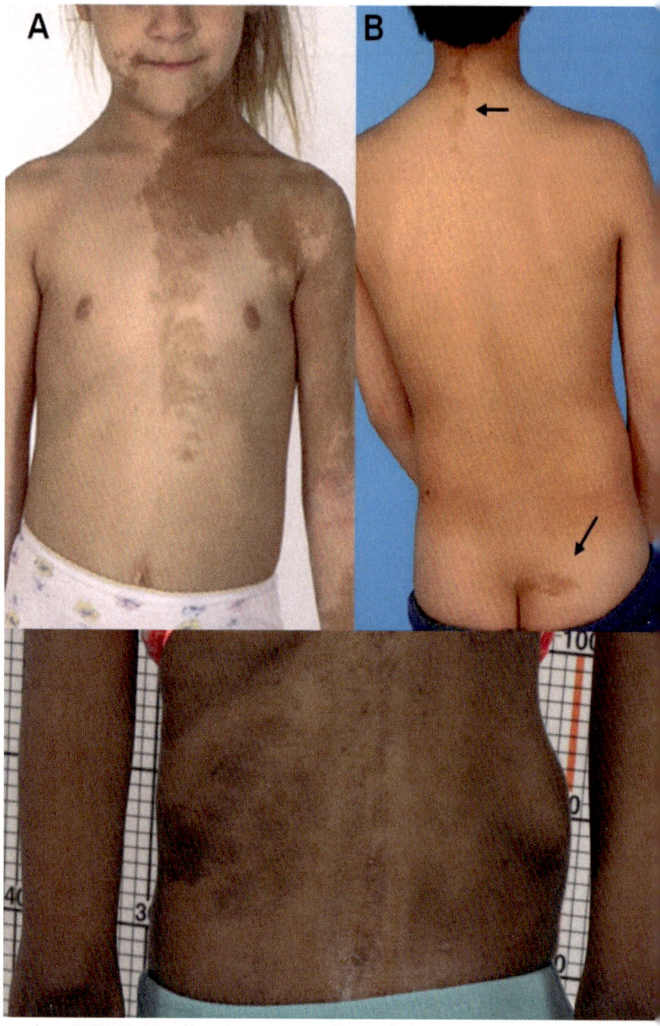

FIGURE 18.1.5 - Unilateral Sharply Contoured Cafe-Au-Lait Spots

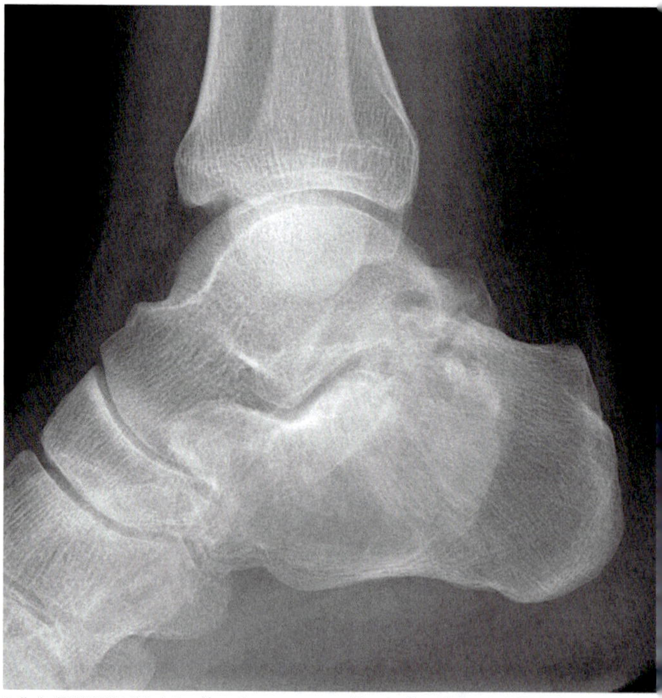

FIGURE 18.1.6 - X-ray: Central Hyperlucency

III. Benign Pubertal Variants
   A. Precocious thelarche: isolated breast development without other secondary sex characteristics
   B. Precocious pubarche: isolated pubic hair development without other secondary sex characteristics
   C. Precocious menarche: isolated initiation of menses without other secondary sex characteristics

IV. Obesity-Related Precocious Puberty
   A. Central pathophysiology: obesity increases leptin → leptin increases GnRH secretion → increased FSH/LH
   B. Peripheral pathophysiology: obesity induces insulin resistance → compensatory hyperinsulinemia → precocious puberty
   C. Insulin: stimulates aromatase in adipocytes and androgen production by adrenal glands and inhibits SHBG synthesis by liver

V. Delayed Puberty
   A. Definition: absent or incompletely formed secondary sex characteristics by age 14 in boys and age 13 in girls
   B. Physiological: constitutional growth delay
   C. Pathological
      1. Hypergonadotropic hypogonadism
      2. Hypogonadotropic hypogonadism
      3. Malnutrition
   D. Constitutional growth delay
      1. Delayed puberty and delayed bone age
      2. Short stature
      3. Normal growth velocity
      4. Family history of constitutional growth delay
   E. Management
      1. Reassurance and waiting; normal adult height usually achieved
   F. Pathological delay of puberty
      1. Hypergonadotropic hypogonadism: Turner syndrome, Klinefelter syndrome
      2. Hypogonadotropic hypogonadism: Kallmann syndrome
      3. Malnutrition: kwashiorkor, marasmus

REVIEW QUESTIONS

1. A 7-year-old boy is brought by his mother to the primary care physician for a routine examination. His height is in the 98th percentile for his age. Physical examination shows increased body and facial hair and testicular enlargement. The mother has recently noticed that her son's voice sounds deeper than previously. What is the next best step in management?

   - **The next best step in the management of suspected precocious puberty is to obtain an X-ray of the hand and wrist to evaluate the bone age.**
   - This 7-year-old boy presents with increased body and facial hair, testicular enlargement, and deeper than normal voice.
   - Since these secondary sex characteristics developed before 9 years of age, he might have precocious puberty.
   - If bone age is greater than the patient's

REVIEW QUESTIONS

chronological age, true precocious puberty is likely, and further workup is indicated.

2. An 8-year-old boy is brought to his primary care physician by his father due to rapid growth in height. The patient's parents noticed that he is growing faster than his siblings. Physical examination shows axillary and pubic hair. Testicular enlargement is also noted. His vital signs include blood pressure of 85/65 mmHg, heart rate of 110 beats/min, and respiratory rate of 18 breaths/min. Laboratory findings are significant for a potassium level of 5.5 mEq/L (3.5 - 5 mEq/L). A 24-hour urine 17-hydroxyprogesterone is elevated. What is the best treatment option for this patient?

   - **The best treatment option for this patient is cortisol supplementation, which will decrease ACTH levels as well as adrenal androgen production.**
   - This 8-year-old boy presents with rapid growth in height, axillary and pubic hair, and testicular enlargement.
   - These secondary sex characteristics in a boy less than 9 years of age suggest precocious puberty.
   - This boy also has hypotension and hyperkalemia with increased 24-hour urine 17-hydroxyprogesterone.
   - All these findings and the age of the patient are consistent with the diagnosis of non-classic congenital adrenal hyperplasia due to 21-hydroxylase deficiency.

3. A 15-year-old boy is brought to his primary care physician by his father for a routine examination. His height is at the 4th percentile for his age. Physical examination shows Tanner stage I genitalia and pubic hair. An X-ray of the left wrist and hand shows the bone age of a 12-year-old. The father recalls that he also started his puberty later than his peers. Serum FSH and LH levels are normal. What is the next best step in the management of this patient?

   - **The next best step in the management of the patient with constitutional growth delay is reassurance because he will likely achieve adult height and normal secondary sex characteristics.**
   - This 15-year-old boy presents with a height at the 4th percentile for his age and Tanner stage I pubic hair and genitalia.
   - His bone age is 12 years.
   - This presentation is consistent with delay of growth and puberty.
   - Since his serum FSH and LH levels are normal, and his father also has a history of delayed puberty, this patient's diagnosis is most likely a constitutional delay of growth and puberty.

Pediatrics | Section 3: Glycogen Storage Diseases

I. Von Gierke Disease: General Features
   A. Von Gierke disease: type I glycogen storage disease
   B. Autosomal recessive
   C. Glucose-6-phosphatase deficiency
   D. Impiared gluconeogenesis and glycogenolysis (glucose-6-phosphatase is common for both pathways)
   E. Glycogen accumulation in liver and kidneys

II. Von Gierke Disease: Clinical Presentation
   A. Severe fasting hypoglycemia
   B. Hepatomegaly and renomegaly
   C. Increased lactate
   D. Increased uric acid
   E. Increased triglycerides
   F. Short stature and thin extremities
   G. Doll-like faces with fat cheeks

III. Von Gierke Disease: Management
   A. Frequent oral glucose/cornstarch administration
   B. Avoidance of fructose and galactose

IV. Pompe Disease: General Features
   A. Pompe disease: type II glycogen storage disease
   B. Autosomal recessive
   C. Acid maltase (lysosomal acid alpha-1,4-glucosidase) deficiency
   D. Glycogen accumulation in heart, liver, and muscle

V. Pompe Disease: Clinical Presentation
   A. Hypertrophic cardiomyopathy (most common cause of death)
   B. Hypotonia
   C. Macroglossia
   D. Early death

VI. Pompe Disease: Management
   A. Enzyme replacement therapy with recombinant human acid alpha-glucosidase

VII. Cori Disease: General Features
   A. Cori disease: type III glycogen storage disease
   B. Autosomal recessive
   C. Debranching enzyme deficiency
   D. Glycogenolysis is impaired but gluconeogenesis is intact
   E. Glycogen with abnormal structure accumulated in cells

VIII. Cori Disease: Clinical Presentation
   A. Similar to von Gierke but milder in severity
   B. Fasting hypoglycemia
   C. Normal lactate levels
   D. Possible cardiomyopathy

IX. Cori Disease: Management
   A. High-protein diet with cornstarch supplementation

X. McArdle Disease: General Features
   A. McArdle disease: type V glycogen storage disease
   B. Autosomal recessive
   C. Myophosphorylase (muscle glycogen phosphorylase) deficiency
   D. Muscles cannot break down glycogen into glucose but liver can
   E. Blood glucose levels usually unaffected

XI. McArdle Disease: Clinical Presentation
   A. Muscle cramps and myoglobinuria during exercise
   B. Arrhythmia due to rhabdomyolysis-induced hyperkalemia
   C. Flat venous lactate curve with normal rise in ammonia levels during exercise
   D. Second-wind phenomenon
      1. Initial muscular weakness followed by normalized muscle strength due to increased muscle blood flow

XII. McArdle Disease: Management
   A. Avoidance of strenuous exercise
   B. Sucrose ingestion before exercise
   C. Creatine supplementation
   D. ACE inhibitors

REVIEW QUESTIONS

1. A 3-month-old boy is brought to the primary care physician by his parents because of irritability and sleepiness for the past 2 weeks. The patient was born at 38 weeks gestation via vaginal delivery. He experienced two episodes of tonic-clonic seizures this week several hours after being breastfed. Physical examination shows a liver span of 18 cm in the midclavicular line and bilateral bulging flank masses. Laboratory findings are significant for hyperuricemia, hypertriglyceridemia, and increased lactic acid. His fasting blood glucose is 30 mg/dL (70 - 100 mg/dL). What is the most likely biochemical explanation for severe fasting hypoglycemia in this patient?
    - **The most likely biochemical explanation for severe fasting hypoglycemia in this patient is interrupted glycogenolysis and gluconeogenesis.**
    - This patient presents with irritability and sleepiness.
    - He had two episodes of tonic-clonic seizure several hours after being breastfed, which were most likely due to fasting hypoglycemia.
    - He has hepatomegaly, evidenced by an 18 cm liver span in the midclavicular line.
    - Additionally, he has enlarged kidneys, evidenced by bilateral bulging flank masses.
    - Finally, his laboratory findings are significant for hyperuricemia, hypertriglyceridemia, increased lactic acid levels, and fasting hypoglycemia of 30 mg/dL.
    - All of these findings are consistent with the diagnosis of von Gierke disease.
    - Von Gierke disease is an autosomal recessive type I glycogen storage disease caused by glucose-6-phosphatase deficiency. This enzyme is common for both glycogenolysis and gluconeogenesis.
    - Therefore, the biochemical explanation for severe fasting hypoglycemia in this patient with von Gierke disease is that both glycogenolysis and gluconeogenesis are interrupted.

2. A 16-year-old girl is brought to the emergency department by her mother due to severe muscle cramps and dark urine. She was exercising in the gym when she suddenly felt diffuse muscular pain and an irregular heartbeat. Urinalysis is significant for 3+ red blood cells, but urine microscopy reveals no erythrocytes. Laboratory findings are significant for a creatine kinase level of 2,000 U/L (10 - 70 U/L) and a potassium level of 5.4 mEq/L (3.5 - 5 mEq/L). Similar episodes have happened to her older brother and sister. She intermittently experiences muscle pain after exercise. However, her cramps usually resolve after eating food and having a short period of rest. What is the best explanation for this patient's increased exercise capacity after rest?
    - **The best explanation for this patient's increased exercise capacity after rest is increased muscular blood flow after a short period of rest.**
    - This young patient presents with severe muscle cramps and dark urine.
    - She has an irregular heartbeat.
    - Lab tests show serum creatine kinase of 2,000 U/L and potassium of 5.4 mEq/L.
    - These findings are consistent with rhabdomyolysis.
    - Given her age and the fact that her brother and sister are also affected, she most likely has a genetic disease.
    - This presentation is classic for McArdle disease, an autosomal recessive type V glycogen storage disease caused by myophosphorylase deficiency.
    - According to the patient, she intermittently experiences muscle pain after exercise. After eating a chocolate bar and having a short period of rest, her cramps usually resolve, and she exercises better. This is a "second-wind phenomenon" characteristic of McArdle disease, which is explained by increased muscular blood flow after a short period of rest.

Pediatrics | Section 4: Lysosomal Storage Diseases Part 1

I. Tay-Sachs Disease: General Features
   A. Autosomal recessive
   B. Deficiency of hexosaminidase-A
   C. GM_2 ganglioside no longer converted to GM_3 ganglioside
   D. GM_2 ganglioside builds up in the lysosomes

II. Tay-Sachs Disease: Clinical Presentation
   A. Neurodevelopmental delay
   B. "Cherry-red" spot on the macula due to lipid accumulation in ganglion cell layer
   C. Hyperreflexia
   D. No hepatosplenomegaly (vs. Niemann-Pick disease)
   E. Excessive startle response
   F. Electron microscopy showing "onion skin" lysosomes

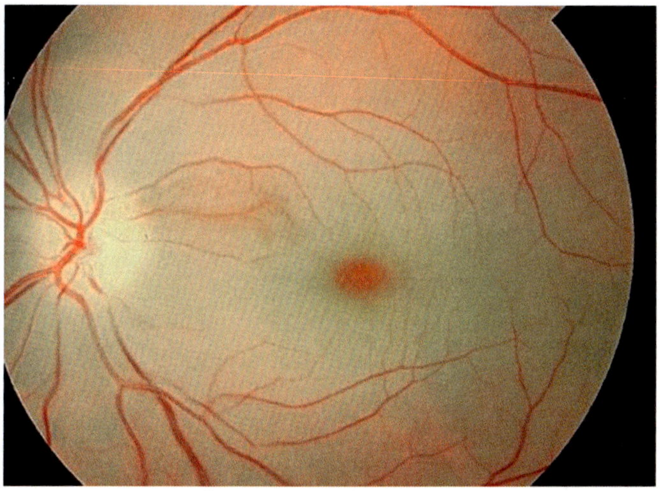

FIGURE 18.1.7 - Fundoscopy: "Cherry-Red" Spot on the Macula

III. Tay-Sachs Disease: Management
   A. Supportive therapy alleviating the symptoms (e.g. antiepileptics)
   B. Poor prognosis

IV. Niemann-Pick Disease: General Features
   A. Autosomal recessive
   B. Sphingomyelinase deficiency (sphingomyelin to ceramide)
   C. Accumulation of sphingomyelin

V. Niemann-Pick Disease: Clinical Presentation
   A. Neurodevelopmental delay
   B. Hepatosplenomegaly (vs. Tay-Sachs)
   C. "Cherry-red" spot on the macula
   D. Foam cells (lipid-laden macrophages)

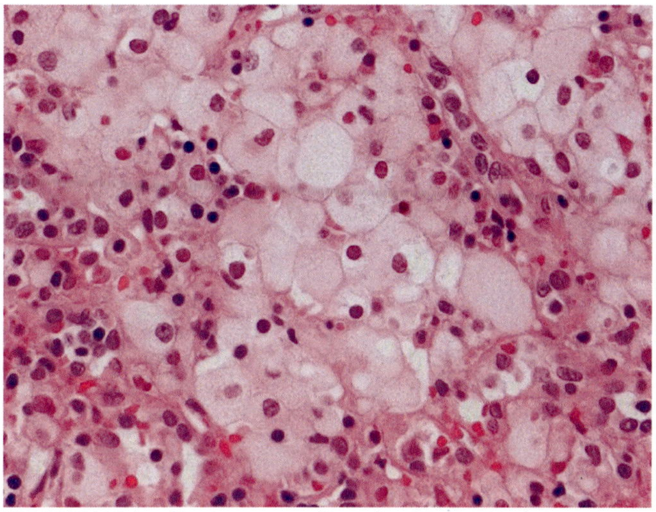

FIGURE 18.1.8 - Light Microscopy: Foam Cells in Niemann-Pick Disease

VI. Niemann-Pick Disease: Management
   A. Physical therapy
   B. Miglustat (not routinely administered)

VII. Fabry Disease: General Features
   A. X-linked recessive
   B. α-galactosidase A (ceramide trihexoside to glucocerebroside)
   C. Accumulation of ceramide trihexoside

VIII. Fabry Disease: Clinical Presentation
   A. Early phase
      1. Peripheral neuropathy (burning hands and feet)
      2. Angiokeratomas
      3. Hypohidrosis
   B. Late phase
      1. Renal failure
      2. Cardiovascular disease

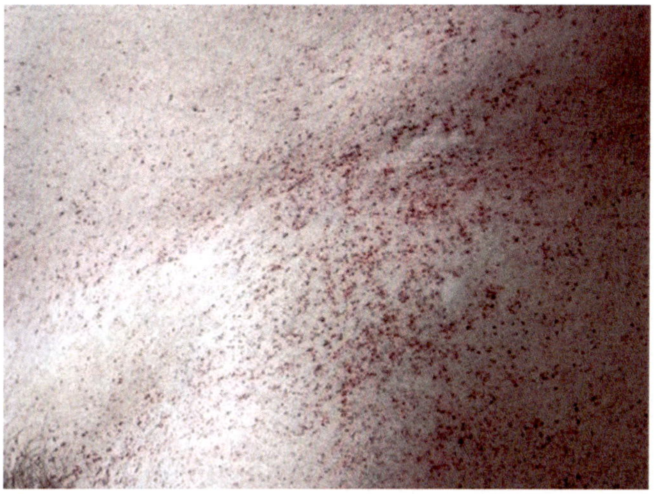

FIGURE 18.1.9 - Angiokeratomas

IX. Fabry Disease: Management
  A. Replacement of α-galactosidase A
  B. Dialysis or renal transplantation for chronic kidney disease
  C. Pharmacological management or heart transplantation for heart failure

X. Metachromatic Leukodystrophy: General Features
  A. Autosomal recessive
  B. Arylsulfatase A (sulfatides into galactocerebroside)
  C. Accumulation of sulfatide (cerebroside sulfate)

XI. Metachromatic Leukodystrophy: Clinical Presentation
  A. Central and peripheral nervous system demyelination
  B. Ataxia
  C. Dementia

XII. Metachromatic Leukodystrophy: Management
  A. Enzyme replacement therapy with arylsulfatase A

REVIEW QUESTIONS

1. A 4-year-old girl is brought to the primary care physician by her parents due to irritability and inability to speak for the last 1 day. She was born at 39 weeks of gestation via vaginal delivery. Physical examination shows hepatosplenomegaly, decreased sensation of the upper and lower extremities, as well as 1+ deep tendon reflexes. Fundoscopic examination shows relative pallor of the retina compared to the normal. What will most likely be seen on light microscopy of this patient's tissue biopsy?

   - **Light microscopy will most likely show foam cells.**
   - This patient presents with irritability and inability to speak for 1 day.
   - Physical exam shows decreased sensation on her upper and lower extremities, hypoactive deep tendon reflexes, and hepatosplenomegaly.
   - Involvement of both the central nervous system and reticuloendothelial system is characteristic of Niemann-Pick disease.
   - Light microscopy of the tissue from the patient with Niemann-Pick disease will show foam cells, that is, sphingomyelin-laden macrophages.

REVIEW QUESTIONS

2. A 5-year-old boy is brought to the primary care physician by his mother due to a rash on his face. She first noticed the skin lesions several months ago, and states they have enlarged since then. The boy complains of burning sensation in his hands and feet. The mother reports that her son does not sweat as much as her other children after playing outdoors. Physical examination shows erythematous papules most prominent on the cheeks. Involvement of which two organ systems is most likely expected in this patient?

   - **The two organ symptoms most likely to be affected in this patient are renal and cardiovascular.**
   - This 5-year-old patient has erythematous papules on the face, most consistent with angiokeratomas; burning sensation in his hands and feet suggestive of peripheral neuropathy; and decreased sweating known as hypohidrosis. This triad is characteristic of the early phase of Fabry disease.
   - The late phase of Fabry disease is characterized by renal failure and cardiovascular disease. Therefore, these two organ systems will most likely be affected later in this patient.

3. A 4-year-old girl is brought to the primary care physician by her parents because she has had difficulty walking for the past 2 years. She used to speak several words, but now she does, her speech is extremely limited. A skin biopsy shows cellular accumulation of cerebroside sulfate. Which enzyme is most likely deficient in this patient?

   - **The enzyme most likely deficient in this patient is arylsulfatase A.**
   - This patient has difficulty walking and regression of speech.
   - Regression of gross motor and verbal skills is suggestive of nervous system involvement.
   - These findings in combination with cellular accumulation of cerebroside sulfate are highly suggestive of metachromatic leukodystrophy.
   - Cerebroside sulfate accumulation in metachromatic leukodystrophy is due to a deficiency of arylsulfatase A enzyme.

Pediatrics | Section 5: Lysosomal Storage Diseases Part 2

I. Krabbe Disease: General Features
   A. Autosomal recessive
   B. Deficiency of galactocerebrosidase (galactosylceramidase)
   C. Accumulation of galactocerebroside and psychosine

II. Krabbe Disease: Clinical Presentation
   A. Destruction of oligodendrocytes
   B. Optic atrophy
   C. Peripheral neuropathy
   D. Globoid cells (macrophages laden with galactocerebroside and psychosine)

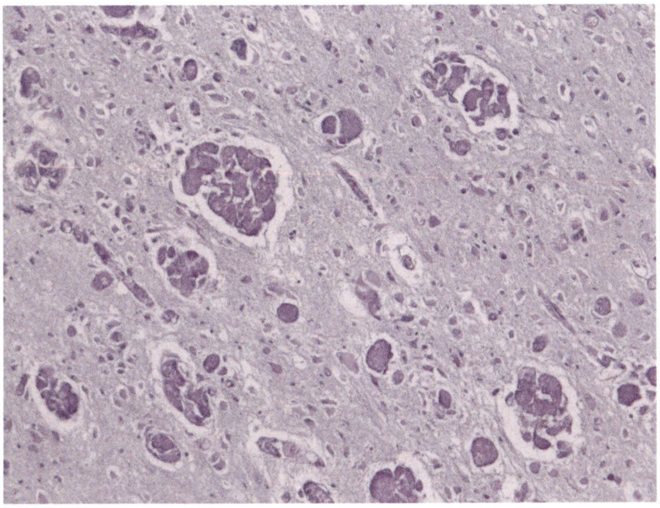

FIGURE 18.1.10 - Light Microscopy: Globoid Cells in Krabbe Disease

III. Krabbe Disease: Management
   A. Supportive treatment
      1. Occupation therapy
      2. Speech therapy

IV. Gaucher Disease: General Features
   A. Autosomal recessive
   B. Glucocerebrosidase (β-glucosidase) deficiency
   C. Accumulation of glucocerebroside

V. Gaucher Disease: Clinical Presentation
   A. Hepatosplenomegaly
   B. Pancytopenia
   C. Osteoporosis
   D. Avascular necrosis of femur
   E. Gaucher cells ("crumpled tissue paper" macrophages)

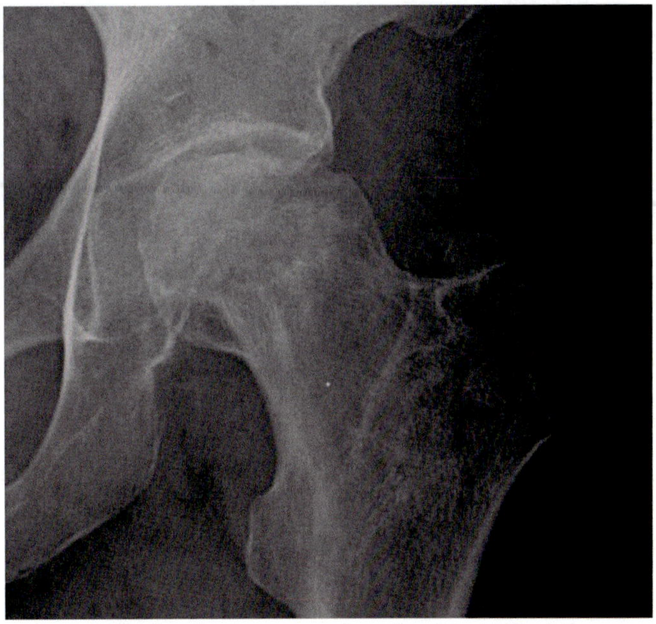

FIGURE 18.1.11 - X-ray of the Hip: Avascular Necrosis of the Femur Head

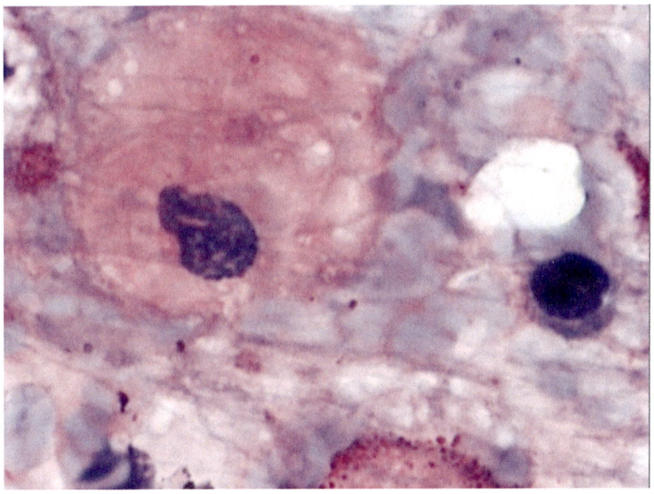

FIGURE 18.1.12 - Light Microscopy: "Crumpled Tissue Paper" Macrophages in Gaucher Disease

VI. Gaucher Disease: Management
   A. Recombinant β-glucosidase

VII. Hurler Syndrome: General Features
   A. Autosomal recessive
   B. α-L-iduronidase deficiency
   C. Accumulation of heparan sulfate and dermatan sulfate

VIII. Hurler Syndrome: Clinical Presentation
   A. Skeletal abnormalities
   B. Airway obstruction
   C. Corneal clouding (vs. Hunter syndrome)
   D. Hepatosplenomegaly

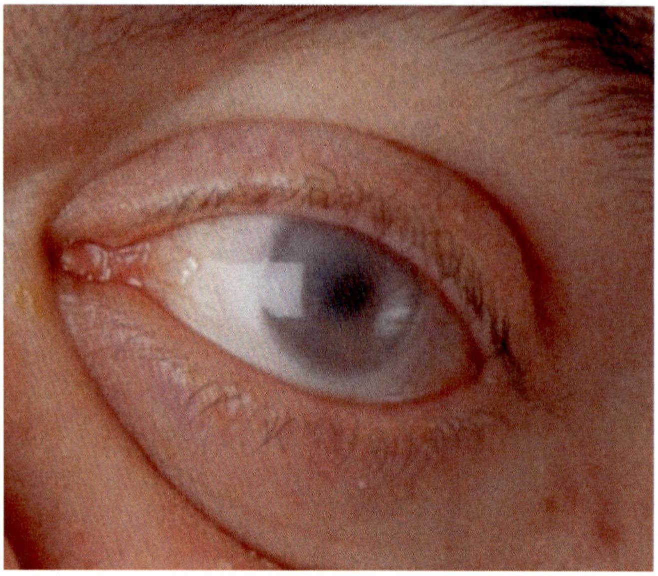

FIGURE 18.1.13 - Corneal Clouding in Hurler Syndrome

IX. Hurler Syndrome: Management
   A. Enzyme replacement therapy with α-L-iduronidase

X. Hunter Syndrome: General Features
   A. X-linked recessive
   B. Deficiency of iduronate-2-sulfatase
   C. Accumulation of heparan sulfate and dermatan sulfate

XI. Hunter Syndrome: Clinical Presentation
   A. Skeletal abnormalities
   B. Hepatosplenomegaly
   C. No corneal clouding
   D. Aggressive behavior

XII. Hunter Syndrome: Management
   A. Enzyme replacement therapy with iduronate-2-sulfatase

REVIEW QUESTIONS

1. A 10-year-old boy is brought to the primary care physician by his parents due to severe fatigue and right hip pain. His fatigue has been present for several years, while his hip pain started 2 weeks ago. He now cannot bear weight on his right leg. Vital signs are unremarkable. Physical examination shows hepatosplenomegaly, tenderness on right hip palpation, and diffuse petechiae. Laboratory findings are significant for hemoglobin of 7 mg/dL (13.5 - 17.5 mg/dL), white blood cell count of 2000 cells/mm^3 (4,500 - 11,000 cells/mm^3), and platelet count of 40,000 cells/mm^3 (150,000 - 400,000 cells/mm^3). X-ray of the right hip shows decreased bone density of the femoral neck consistent with avascular necrosis. Bone marrow biopsy reveals cells with "crumpled tissue paper" appearing cytoplasm. Which of the following is the best treatment option for this patient?

   A. Recombinant sphingomyelinase
   B. Recombinant beta-glucosidase
   C. Systemic chemotherapy
   D. Anti-thymocyte globulin

- **The correct answer is option B.**
- This patient presents with fatigue, right hip pain and is found to be pancytopenic
- X-ray of the right hip shows decreased bone density of the femoral neck consistent with avascular necrosis.
- Bone marrow biopsy shows cells with "crumpled tissue paper" cytoplasm, called Gaucher cells.
- These features are classic for Gaucher disease, an autosomal recessive lysosomal storage disease caused by beta-glucosidase deficiency.
- Option A is incorrect because recombinant sphingomyelinase would be used in Niemann-Pick disease. Niemann-Pick disease presents with hepatosplenomegaly, neurological impairment, and the "cherry-red spot" on the macula. This patient has no neurological abnormalities.
- Option C is incorrect because systemic chemotherapy can be in multiple forms of cancer but is not indicated in Gaucher disease.
- Option D is incorrect because anti-thymocyte globulin is used in primary aplastic anemia. Although this patient has pancytopenia characteristic of aplastic anemia, he also has avascular necrosis and hepatosplenomegaly, and the bone marrow biopsy shows "crumpled tissue paper" macrophages. These findings are not characteristic of aplastic anemia.

Pediatrics | Section 6: Inborn Errors of Metabolism

I. Classic Galactosemia (autosomal recessive): General Features
   - A. Galactose-1-phosphate uridyltransferase (GALT) deficiency
   - B. Inability to convert galactose-1-phosphate to glucose-1-phosphate
   - C. Galactosemia and galactosuria (reducing substance in the urine)
   - D. Excess galactose is converted to galactitol

II. Classic Galactosemia: Clinical Presentation
   - A. Clinical features
     1. Infantile cataracts; nausea and vomiting
     2. *E.coli* sepsis; hepatomegaly; jaundice
     3. More severe than galactokinase deficiency
     4. Galactokinase deficiency: absence of liver damage (Galactose-1-phosphate does not accumulate in liver)

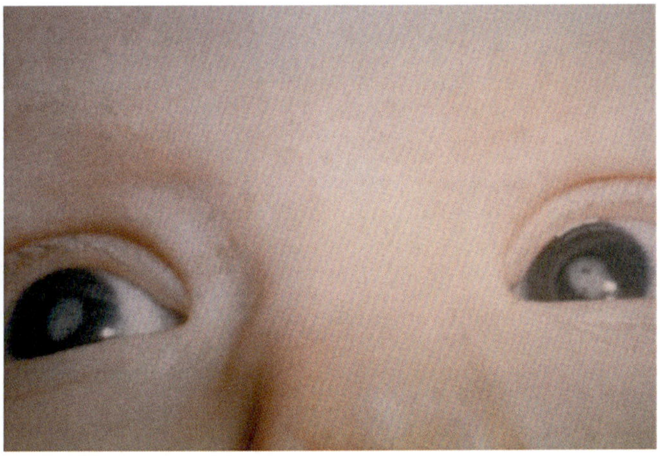

See page for author, Public domain, via Wikimedia Commons

FIGURE 18.1.14 - Infant with Bilateral Cataracts

III. Classic Galactosemia: Diagnosis
   - A. Newborn screening
   - B. Laboratory findings:
     1. ↑ bilirubin, ↑ AST/ALT, ↓ glucose
   - C. Urinalysis:
     1. Reducing substance in urine (galactose)
   - D. Measurement of GALT enzyme activity in red blood cells
   - E. DNA testing for GALT gene mutation

IV. Classic Galactosemia: Management
   - A. Avoidance of:
     1. Galactose
     2. Lactose (galactose and glucose)

V. Phenylketonuria: General Features
   - A. Autosomal recessive
   - B. Classic PKU: phenylalanine hydroxylase deficiency
   - C. Tyrosine becomes an essential amino acid
   - D. Excess phenylalanine: phenyl ketones (phenylacetate, phenyllactate, phenylpyruvate)

VI. Phenylketonuria: Clinical Presentation
   - A. Intellectual disability (due to deficiency of several neurotransmitters)
   - B. Microcephaly
   - C. Seizures
   - D. Musty body odor (due to phenyl ketones)
   - E. Fair skin (due to decreased melanin production)

VII. Phenylketonuria: Diagnosis
   - A. Screening 2 - 3 days after birth (normal results at birth due to effect of maternal enzyme)
   - B. Quantitative amino acid analysis
   - C. Measurement of phenyl ketones in blood or urine
   - D. Genetic testing (not always performed)

VIII. Phenylketonuria: Management
   - A. Increase tyrosine and decrease phenylalanine in diet
   - B. Supplement tetrahydrobiopterin
   - C. Avoid aspartame (artificial sweetener containing phenylalanine)

IX. Homocystinuria: General Features
   - A. Autosomal recessive disease causing homocysteine accumulation
   - B. Causes
     1. Cystathionine synthase deficiency (homocysteine → cystathionine)
     2. Decreased affinity of cystathionine synthase to pyridoxal phosphate
     3. Methionine synthase deficiency (homocysteine → methionine)
     4. Methylenetetrahydrofolate reductase deficiency (DHF → THF)

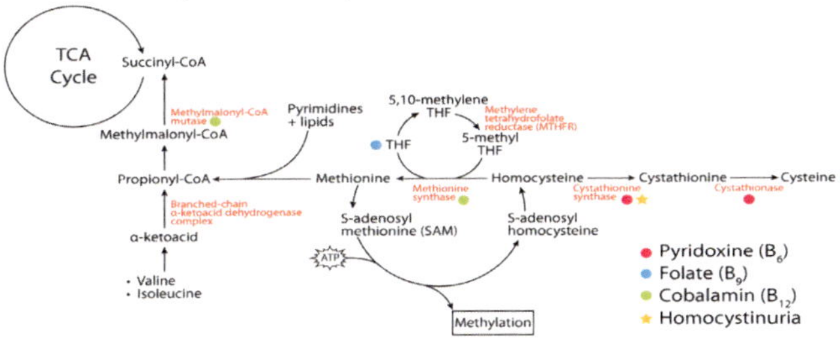

FIGURE 18.1.15 - Pathways of Homocysteine Metabolism

X. Homocystinuria: Clinical Presentation
   - A. Osteoporosis
   - B. Marfanoid habitus (tall stature, long wingspan)
   - C. Downward and inward displacement of lens (vs. Marfan)
   - D. Intellectual disability (vs. Marfan)
   - E. Stroke and myocardial infarction
   - F. Megaloblastic anemia and joint hyperlaxity

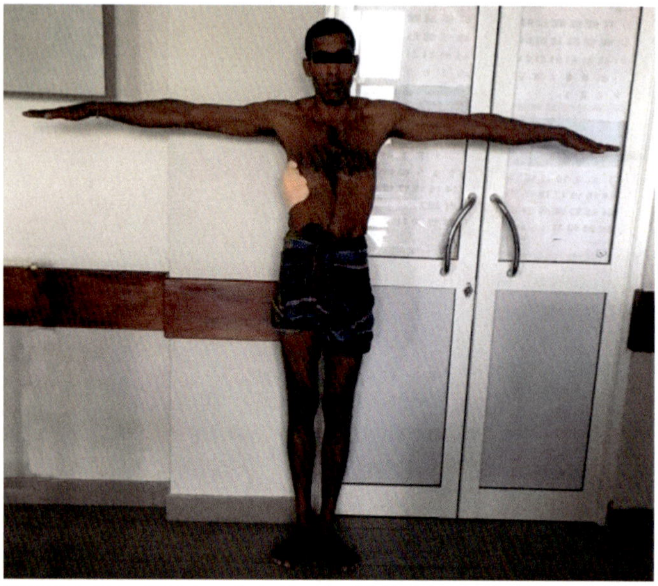

FIGURE 18.1.16 - Marfanoid Habitus

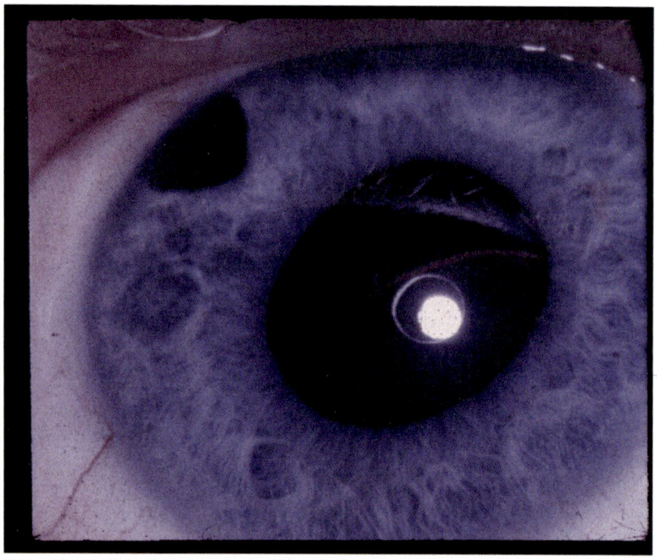

FIGURE 18.1.17 - Homocystinuria

XI. Homocystinuria: Diagnosis
    A. Measurement of homocysteine in urine or blood

XII. Homocystinuria: Management
    A. B_6, B_9, and B_{12} to lower homocysteine levels
    B. Anticoagulants or antiplatelets to prevent thrombotic complications (e.g. myocardial infarction, stroke)

XIII. Cystinuria: General Features
    A. Autosomal recessive condition leading to decreased reabsorption of **C**ystine, **O**rnithine, **L**ysine, and **A**rginine

XIV. Cystinuria: Clinical Presentation
    A. Recurrent kidney stones starting from early age

XV. Cystinuria: Diagnosis
    A. Cystine crystals have hexagonal shape on urine microscopy
    B. Urinary sodium-cyanide nitroprusside test (red-purple hue)
    C. Proton nuclear magnetic resonance spectroscopy of urine

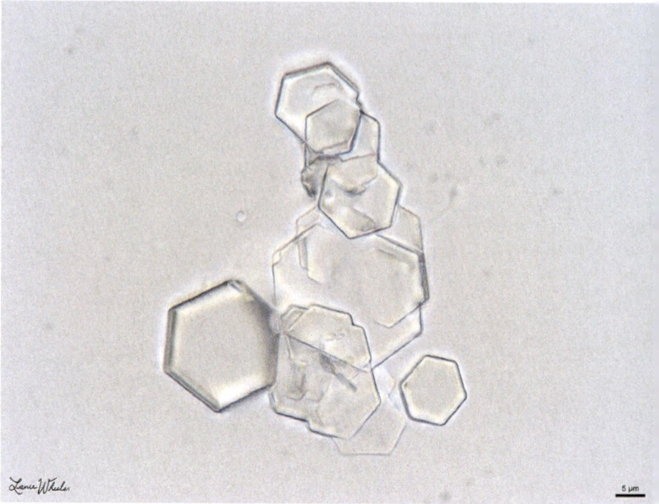

FIGURE 18.1.18 - Cystine Crystals in Urine

XVI. Cystinuria: Management
    A. Urine alkalinization
        1. Potassium citrate
        2. Acetazolamide
    B. Chelating agents
        1. Penicillamine

REVIEW QUESTIONS

1. A 1-month-old girl is brought to the emergency department by her parents due to severe nausea and vomiting for the last 2 weeks. Her symptoms worsen every time she is breastfed. She was born at 37 weeks of gestation via cesarean delivery. The physical examination shows hepatosplenomegaly and jaundice. Fundoscopic examination shows bilateral opacification of the lens. Systemic infection with which microbe is likely to develop in this patient?

    - **This patient is at an increased risk for *E.coli*.**
    - This patient presents with severe nausea, vomiting, jaundice, hepatosplenomegaly, and infantile cataracts, as evidenced by bilateral opacification of the lens.
    - Her symptoms worsen every time she is breastfed.
    - Breast milk contains lactose, a disaccharide composed of galactose and glucose.
    - This presentation is consistent with classic galactosemia.

REVIEW QUESTIONS

2. A 3-day-old boy is evaluated for tonic-clonic seizures. He was born at 41 weeks of gestation via cesarean delivery. He has a musty body odor, and physical examination shows fair skin, hair, and microcephaly. Which amino acid should be supplemented in this patient's diet?

- **The amino acid Tyrosine should be supplemented in this boy's diet.**
- He presents with seizures, a musty odor, microcephaly, and fair complexion.
- All these findings point towards the diagnosis of phenylketonuria (PKU).
- Phenylketonuria is an autosomal recessive disorder most commonly caused by deficiency of phenylalanine hydroxylase.
- Therefore, phenylalanine is no longer converted to tyrosine.

3. A 10-year-old girl is brought to the primary care physician by her parents for follow-up after a deep venous thrombosis 3 months ago. She has a history of diagnosed intellectual disability. Physical examination shows excessive joint flexibility, tall stature, and downward displacement of the lens. The physician suspected homocystinuria. What are the similarities and differences in the clinical features of homocystinuria and Marfan syndrome?

Homocystinuria	Marfan Syndrome
Tall stature	Tall stature
Pectus deformity	Pectus deformity
Joint hyperlaxity	Joint hyperlaxity
Arachnodactyly	Arachnodactyly
Skin hyperelasticity	Skin hyperelasticity
Scoliosis	Scoliosis
Autosomal recessive	Autosomal dominant
Intellectual disability	Normal intellect
Downward and inward lens dislocation	Upward lens dislocation
Thrombosis	Aortic root dilation
Megaloblastic anemia and fair complexion	No megaloblastic anemia and fair complexion

TABLE 18.1.3 - Homocystinuria and Marfan Syndrome Characteristics

1. A 15-year-old boy is brought to the primary care physician by his mother for a follow-up visit after ST-elevation myocardial infarction 4 weeks ago. He was diagnosed with intellectual disability at 3 years old. He is very tall with a slender build, long fingers, and a large wing span. Vital signs include temperature of 96.8° F (36° C), blood pressure of 125/70 mmHg, heart rate of 92 beats/min, and respiratory rate of 14 breaths/min. Physical exam shows kyphoscoliosis and fundoscopic examination shows downward and inward lens displacement. Which of the following is the next best step in the diagnosis of this patient?

   A. Measurement of serum homocysteine levels
   B. DNA testing for *FBN*1 gene mutation
   C. Urine sodium cyanide-nitroprusside test
   D. Measurement of serum B_{12} levels

- **The correct answer is option A.**
- This young patient presents with an early ST-elevation myocardial infarction, intellectual disability, and marfanoid habitus including long fingers, tall stature, and a large wing span.
- Additionally, the physical exam shows downward and inward lens displacement, as well as severe kyphoscoliosis.
- All of these findings suggest the diagnosis of homocystinuria.
- The best next step in diagnosing homocystinuria is measuring serum homocysteine levels.
- Option B is incorrect because DNA testing for *FBN*1 gene mutation is used to diagnose Marfan syndrome rather than homocystinuria.
- Although these two conditions are similar, Marfan syndrome is not characterized by intellectual disability and myocardial infarction.
- Option C is incorrect because the urine sodium cyanide-nitroprusside test is used to diagnose cystinuria rather than homocystinuria.
- Option D is incorrect because although the patients with homocystinuria should be supplemented with vitamin B_{12}, measurement of serum B_{12} levels is not necessary for diagnosis.

Pediatrics | Section 7: Complications in the Newborn Period - APGAR Scores, and Extracranial Injuries

I. APGAR Score
   A. Standardized clinical assessment of newborns
   B. Performed at one and five minutes
   C. Five components, each can be scored from 0 to 2
   D. Do not let calculating an APGAR score delay resuscitation
   E. Not a long-term prognostic tool
   F. Maximum score: 10
   G. Minimum score: 0
   H. Interpretation
      1. Scores between 7 and 10 are normal
      2. Scores between 4 and 6 are moderately abnormal
      3. Scores between 0 and 3 are abnormal

Condition	Scoring
Appearance (skin color)	- 0 points: blue - 1 point: acrocyanosis - 2 points: pink body and extremities
Pulse	- 0 points: no pulse - 1 point: < 100 bpm - 2 points: ≥ 100 bpm
Grimace (irritability with tactile stimulation)	- 0 points: none - 1 point: grimace - 2 points: cry or withdrawal
Activity (muscle tone)	- 0 points: no movement, limp - 1 point: some flexion - 2 points: active motion
Respiration	- 0 points: none - 1 point: weak cry, irregular or slow breathing - 2 points: regular breathing, strong cry

TABLE 18.1.4 - APGAR Score

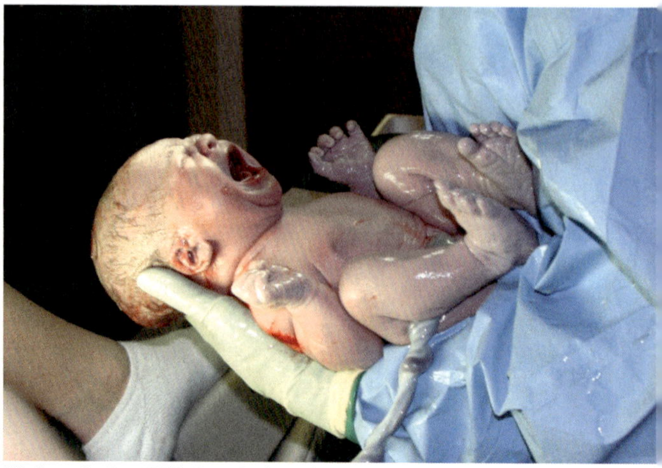

FIGURE 18.1.19 - Acrocyanosis

II. Extracranial Injuries: Caput Succedaneum
   A. Secondary to prolonged engagement of the head in the birth canal or vacuum extraction
   B. Diffuse, edematous swelling that can cross suture lines
   C. Benign condition that resolves in a few days

III. Extracranial Injuries: Cephalohematoma
   A. Subperiosteal collection of blood secondary to rupture of blood vessels beneath the periosteum
   B. Swelling that does not cross suture lines
   C. May rarely expand in first few days
   D. Resolves over the course of weeks
   E. Can lead to neonatal jaundice

IV. Extracranial Injuries: Subgaleal Hemorrhage
   A. Accumulation of blood between the periosteum of the skull and the epicranial aponeurosis
   B. Due to injury of the emissary veins during delivery
   C. Diffuse, fluctuant swelling of the head that can cross suture lines
      1. Can extend to the neck
   D. May expand in hours to days after delivery
   E. Can result in extensive blood loss, hemorrhagic shock, and death

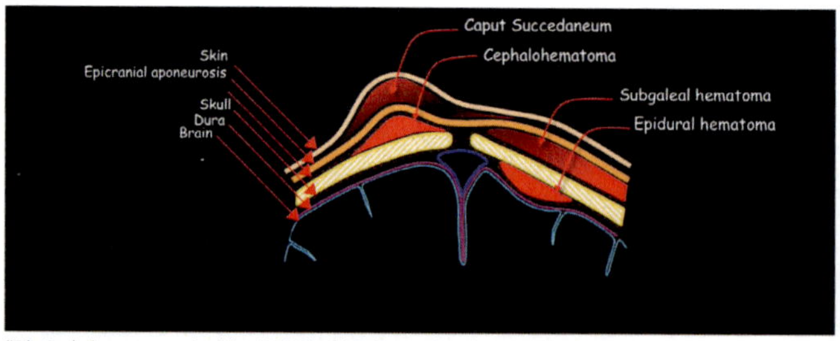

FIGURE 18.1.20 - Extracranial Injuries

Condition	Etiology	Key Features
Caput succedaneum	- Prolonged engagement of fetal head in birth canal - Vacuum extraction	- Can cross suture lines - Resolves in a few days
Cephalohematoma	- Rupture of blood vessels beneath the periosteum	- Does not cross suture lines - Resolves in a few weeks
Subgaleal hemorrhage	- Accumulation of blood between periosteum and aponeurosis - Rupture of emissary veins	- Diffuse, fluctuant swelling of head - Can result in extensive blood loss and hemorrhagic shock

TABLE 18.1.5 - Extracranial Injuries

REVIEW QUESTIONS

1. A baby boy is born to a 25-year-old mother at 38 weeks gestation. He is assessed by the pediatrician at 1 minute following vaginal delivery. Physical examination shows a pink head and trunk with blue extremities. He cries vigorously and pulls away when stimulated. He actively moves the upper and lower extremities. His heart rate is 95 beats/min. What is the correct interpretation of this patient's Apgar score?

   - **This patient's Apgar score is normal.**
   - This patient has acrocyanosis; therefore, he gets 1 point for appearance.
   - Vigorous cry earns him 2 points for respiration.
   - The fact that he pulls away when stimulated earns him 2 points for grimace.
   - Additionally, he gets 2 points for active upper and lower extremities movement.
   - Finally, the heart rate is less than 100 beats/min, which earns him 1 point for pulse.
   - Therefore, an Apgar score for this particular patient is 8. Apgar scores from 7 to 10 are considered normal.

2. A baby girl was born 5 hours ago to a 32-year-old mother with poorly controlled type I diabetes mellitus. The neonate was delivered vaginally. There was prolonged second stage of labor due to fetal macrosomia and cephalopelvic disproportion. Apgar scores of the infant were 8 and 9 at 1 and 5 minutes, respectively. Physical examination shows a bulge on the left side of the head that does not cross the sagittal suture line. How does this patient's condition differ from caput succedaneum and subgaleal hemorrhage?

   - **First, caput succedaneum is the soft tissue swelling between the skin and the epicranial aponeurosis of the scalp, and subgaleal hemorrhage is bleeding between epicranial aponeurosis and the outer periosteum. In contrast, cephalohematoma is bleeding between the outer periosteum and the skull bone.**
   - **Secondly, caput succedaneum and subgaleal hemorrhage cross the suture line, while cephalohematoma does not.**
   - **Finally, caput succedaneum and cephalohematoma have good prognosis because swelling of bleeding is confined within the closed space. In contrast, subgaleal hemorrhage can result in significant volume depletion and subsequent jaundice due to red blood cell breakdown.**
   - This patient had macrosomia, possibly due to poorly controlled maternal type I diabetes mellitus.
   - Macrosomia resulted in cephalopelvic disproportion, resulting in a prolonged second stage of labor.
   - Complicated delivery is the likely cause of the bulge on the left side of this patient's head.
   - The bulge does not cross the sagittal suture line. This description is most consistent with cephalohematoma.

Pediatrics | Section 8: Complications in the Newborn Period - Neonatal Jaundice

I. Neonatal Jaundice
   A. Usually a benign condition
   B. If severe, may result in kernicterus
      1. Bilirubin encephalopathy due to deposition of unconjugated bilirubin in basal ganglia and brainstem
      2. Leads to chronic neurologic deficits such as cerebral paresis, hearing impairment, movement disorders, intellectual and developmental disabilities
   C. Important history
      1. Gestational age
      2. Birth injuries such as caput succedaneum or cephalohematoma
      3. Maternal blood type and infectious disease workup
      4. Family history
   D. Physical exam
      1. Jaundice spreads in a cephalocaudal pattern
      2. Look for cephalohematoma, bruising, hepatomegaly
      3. Stool color
      4. Signs of dehydration or sepsis
      5. Compare current weight to birth weight

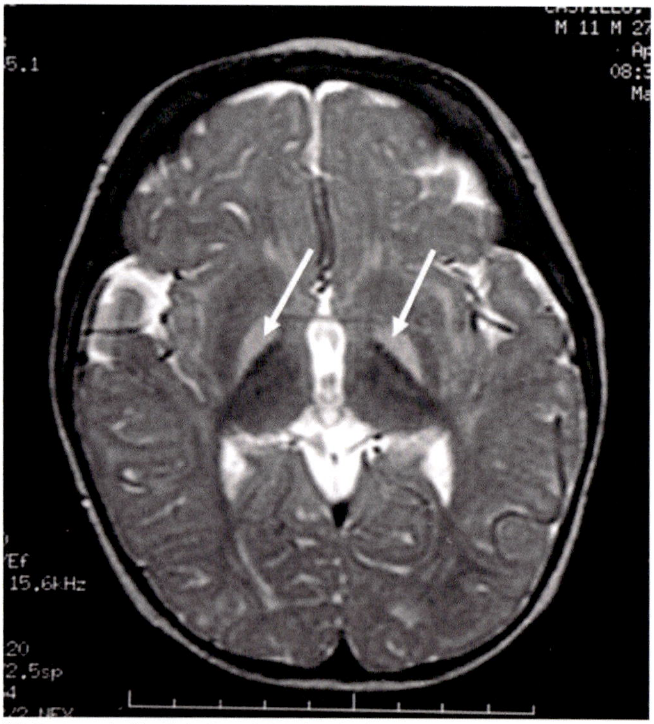

FIGURE 18.1.21 - MRI of the Brain: Bilateral Hyperintensities in the Basal Ganglia (Kernicterus)

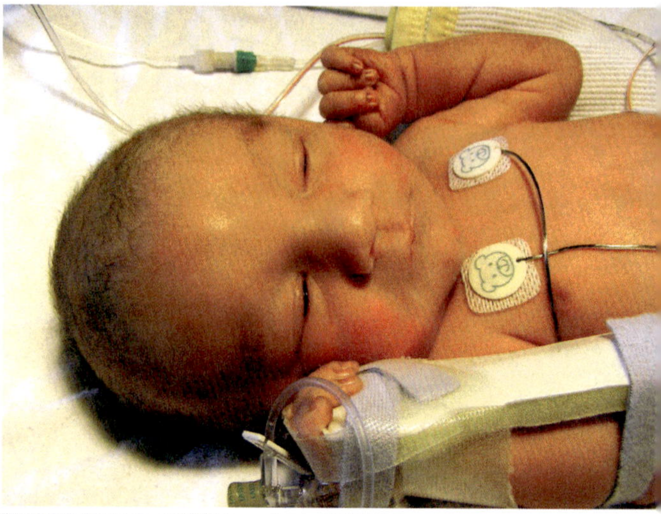

FIGURE 18.1.22 - Jaundice

II. Neonatal Jaundice: Unconjugated Hyperbilirubinemia
   A. Physiologic jaundice
      1. Starts after day one, peaks at days 3 - 4, resolves by days 7 - 10
      2. Due to short lifespan of fetal red blood cells, immature liver enzymes, and increased enterohepatic circulation
      3. Clinical diagnosis
      4. Total bilirubin levels at peak should be < 18 mg/dL in most infants
   B. Breastfeeding jaundice
      1. Onset in first week of life
      2. Due to decreased milk intake leading to dehydration
      3. Hypovolemia → increased enterohepatic circulation → hyperbilirubinemia
      4. Pay close attention to urine and stool output, weight
      5. Weight loss > 10% may need supplementation with formula
   C. Breast milk jaundice
      1. Later onset in second to third weeks of life
      2. Unclear etiology; thought to be due to high levels of β-glucuronidase
      3. Continue to monitor the infant to ensure that bilirubin remains unconjugated and levels do not increase
   D. Hemolytic disease
      1. Typically presents within first 24 hours of life
      2. Can be due to ABO or Rh incompatibility
      3. Ranges from mild disease with jaundice to severe anemia
      4. Lab results will reveal evidence of blood group incompatibility

E. Gilbert syndrome
   1. Benign autosomal recessive condition
   2. Deficiency of UDP-glucuronosyltransferase (UGT) activity
   3. Mild, fluctuating non-hemolytic jaundice that will continue into adulthood
   4. Present at birth, but frequently manifests in adolescence
   5. Exacerbated by certain drugs, fasting, stress
F. Crigler-Najjar syndrome
   1. Due to absence (type 1) or near complete absence (type 2) of UGT
   2. Type 1 is fatal due to the complete inability to eliminate bilirubin leading to
   3. kernicterus
   4. Bilirubin levels may be greater than 50 mg/dL in severe cases
G. Management
   1. Indications based on Bhutani nomogram
H. Phototherapy
   1. Converts unconjugated bilirubin in the skin to water-soluble forms that can be excreted
   2. Goal bilirubin < 15 mg/dL
I. Exchange transfusion
   1. Total bilirubin > 20 mg/dL
   2. Bilirubin encephalopathy, inadequate response to phototherapy, rapid rise in the bilirubin level
   3. Matched blood will be exchanged through an umbilical catheter

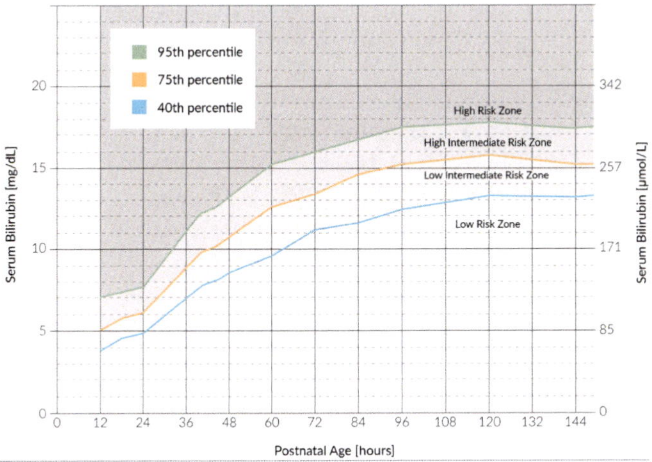

FIGURE 18.1.23 - Bhutani Nomogram

III. Neonatal Jaundice: Conjugated Hyperbilirubinemia
A. Secondary to failure of bile excretion
   1. Can be due to physical obstructions, TORCH infections, cystic fibrosis, metabolic diseases
B. Conjugated hyperbilirubinemia is never physiologic
C. Biliary atresia
   1. Most common surgical cause of neonatal cholestasis
   2. Obliteration or fibrosis of the biliary system
   3. Neonatal jaundice presenting later at 3-6 weeks of life
   4. Associated with acholic stools and dark urine
   5. Diagnosed with ultrasound showing atretic, small, irregular gallbladder
D. Choledochal cysts
   1. Congenital cysts may be due to maldevelopment of the biliary system
   2. May present in infancy as obstructive jaundice with an abdominal mass
   3. Classic triad: abdominal pain, jaundice, abdominal mass
   4. Diagnosed with ultrasound; some may be noticed prenatally
E. Management
   1. Removal of the obstruction
   2. Biliary atresia: Hepatoportoenterostomy (Kasai procedure) connects the liver to the small intestine allowing bile drainage
   3. If there is liver cirrhosis, patient will require transplant

Condition	Etiology	Key Features
Physiologic jaundice	- Short life span fetal RBCs - Immature liver enzymes	- Starts after day one - Peaks at days 3 - 4
Breastfeeding jaundice	- Due to decreased milk intake leading to dehydration	- Onset in first week of life - Associated with signs of dehydration - Infant may lose more than > 10% birth weight
Breast milk jaundice	- Product in milk leads to hyperbilirubinemia	- Later onset at 2 - 3 weeks in breastfed infants
Hemolytic disease	- Due to ABO or Rh incompatibility	- Presents in first 24 hours of life - Labs show blood group incompatibility
Gilbert disease	- Autosomal recessive deficiency of UGT	- Benign, mild, fluctuating jaundice - Exacerbated by drugs, stress - Typically manifests in adolescence
Crigler-Najjar syndrome	- Absence or near complete absence of UGT	- Type 1 is fatal - Leads to kernicterus
Biliary atresia	- Obliteration of fibrosis of biliary system	- Presents at 3 - 6 weeks of life - Acholic stools and dark urine
Choledochal cyst	- Congenital cysts due to maldevelopment of biliary system	- Obstructive jaundice with abdominal mass

TABLE 18.1.6 - Neonatal Jaundice

REVIEW QUESTIONS

1. A 5-day-old boy is brought to the primary care physician by his mother who reports yellow discoloration of her son's skin. The patient was born at 39 weeks gestation via vaginal delivery. His birth weight was 6.6 lbs (3,000 g), and his current weight is 5.5 lbs (2,500 g). The mother is blood type A positive, while her son is blood type B positive. In addition to jaundice, the mother notes that the patient is less active. He has had 3 wet diapers during the last day. Vital signs include a temperature of 98.6° F (37° C), blood pressure of 55/40 mmHg, heart rate of 175 beats/min, and respiratory rate of 50 breaths/min. He is breastfed every 5 to 6 hours. His total bilirubin level is 10 mg/dL (< 5 mg/dL) with a direct fraction of 0.2 mg/dL (0-0.3 mg/dL). Which of the following is the next best step in the management of this patient?

   A. Encourage more frequent breastfeeds
   B. Initiate phototherapy
   C. Initiate exchange transfusion
   D. Reassurance

- **The correct answer is option A.**
- This baby boy presents with jaundice, hypotension, and weight loss.
- Additionally, he lost more than 10% of his birth weight.
- Normally, the number of wet diapers within the first week of life should be equal to the number of days since birth. For example, a 5-day-old neonate should have at least 5 wet diapers.
- All of these findings are consistent with severe dehydration.
- This is also supported by the fact that he is breastfed every 5 to 6 hours. Normally, a neonate should be breastfed every 2 to 3 hours.
- Therefore, the most likely diagnosis of this patient is breastfeeding jaundice.
- Breastfeeding jaundice is caused by insufficient breastfeeding. Decreased bowel movement frequency causes more indirect bilirubin retention, resulting in jaundice. Therefore, the best next step in the management of this patient is to encourage the mother to breastfeed more frequently.
- Options B and C are incorrect because phototherapy and exchange transfusion are necessary for severe indirect hyperbilirubinemia. This patient, on the other hand, has mild hyperbilirubinemia, marked by total bilirubin levels of < 10.
- Option D is incorrect because reassurance would be appropriate for physiological jaundice. This patient has explicit signs of dehydration, making physiologic jaundice less likely.

Pediatrics | Section 9: Complications in the Newborn Period - Respiratory Pathologies

I. Respiratory Distress Syndrome
   A. Respiratory distress secondary to surfactant deficiency
      1. Results in high alveolar surface tension
      2. Low lung compliance and volume with alveolar collapse
   B. Most common in extremely preterm infants
   C. Severity is related to gestational age
   D. Risk factors: prematurity, maternal diabetes, cesarean delivery
   E. Clinical presentation
      1. Extremely preterm infant with signs of respiratory distress such as grunting or cyanosis
   F. Diagnosis: chest X-ray showing reticulogranular "ground-glass" densities, low lung volume, air bronchograms
   G. Management
      1. Antenatal steroids decrease the risk
      2. Prophylactic surfactant at birth in high-risk infants, or as rescue therapy
      3. CPAP
      4. Mechanical ventilation if in respiratory failure
      5. Monitor for symptoms of a pneumothorax while ventilating
   H. Long-term complications
      1. Retinopathy of prematurity: elevated levels of oxygen lead to pathological neovascularization
      2. Bronchopulmonary dysplasia: chronic lung disease due to prolonged mechanical ventilation and oxygen exposure

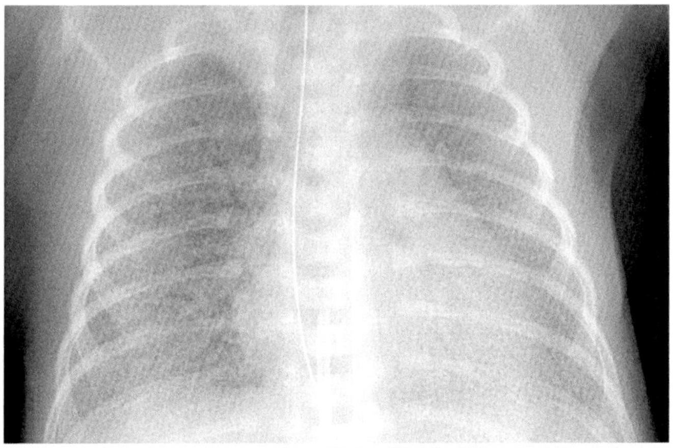

FIGURE 18.1.24 - X-ray of the Chest: Reticulogranular "Ground-Glass" Densities and Air Bronchograms in Respiratory Distress Syndrome

II. Transient Tachypnea of the Newborn
   A. Benign parenchymal lung disorder
   B. Pulmonary edema due to delayed clearance and resorption of fetal alveolar fluid
   C. Usually present in late preterm or term infants
   D. Risk factors: cesarean delivery and maternal diabetes
   E. Clinical presentation: neonate in respiratory distress
      1. Grunting, increased work of breathing, hypoxia
   F. Diagnosis
      1. Clinical diagnosis
      2. Chest X-ray: fluid in interlobar fissures, increased lung volume, potential pleural effusions
   G. Management
      1. Supportive
      2. May require oxygen therapy, CPAP

III. Meconium Aspiration Syndrome
   A. Occurs when neonate aspirates meconium they have passed in utero
   B. Risk factors
      1. Post-term infant
      2. Nonreassuring fetal heart rate tracings during labor/delivery
      3. Placental insufficiency
      4. Oligohydramnios
      5. Maternal hypertension, diabetes, infection
   C. Clinical features
      1. Respiratory distress immediately after birth (tachypnea, increased work of breathing, hypoxia)
      2. Meconium stained amniotic fluid
      3. Rales/rhonchi on auscultation of lungs
   D. Diagnosis
      1. Chest X-ray: increased lung volumes, asymmetric patchy opacities, potential pleural effusions
   E. Management
      1. Supportive care with oxygen and ventilation
      2. May require inhaled nitric oxide or administration of surfactant
      3. Monitor for signs of pneumothorax due to ball-valve effect

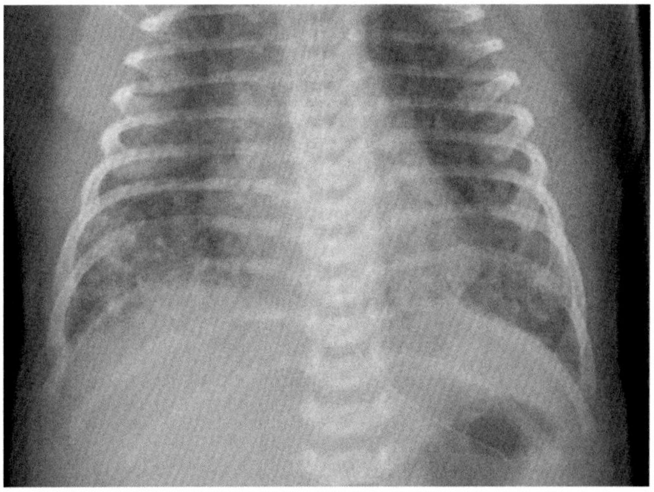

FIGURE 18.1.25 - X-ray of the Chest: Asymmetric, Patchy Opacities in Meconium Aspiration Syndrome

Condition	Etiology	Key Features
Respiratory distress syndrome	- Deficiency of surfactant in preterm infants	- CXR: reticulonodular "ground-glass" opacities and low lung volume
Transient tachypnea of the newborn	- Delayed clearance and resorption of fetal alveolar fluid	- CXR: fluid in interlobar fissures, increased lung volume - Late preterm or term infant - Increased risk in cesarean delivery
Meconium aspiration syndrome	- Neonate aspirates meconium that they passed in utero	- CXR: asymmetric patchy opacities, increased lung volumes - Post-term infants, infants with non-reassuring fetal heart rate tracings during delivery

TABLE 18.1.7 - Neonatal Respiratory Pathologies

REVIEW QUESTIONS

1. A baby boy is evaluated for increased respiratory rate. He was born to a 29-year-old mother 5 hours ago via cesarean delivery. Apgar scores were 9 and 9 at 1 and 5 minutes, respectively. Vital signs include a temperature of 98.6° F (37° C), blood pressure of 70/50 mmHg, heart rate of 150 beats/min, and respiratory rate of 70 breaths/min. Chest X-ray shows perihilar linear streaks consistent with fluid in the interlobar fissures. How does this patient's condition differ from respiratory distress syndrome and meconium aspiration syndrome?

- **First, transient tachypnea of the newborn is caused by inadequate resorption of alveolar fluid; neonatal respiratory distress syndrome is caused by insufficient surfactant production; while meconium aspiration syndrome is caused by meconium-induced chemical irritation of the lungs.**
- **Additionally, transient tachypnea of the newborn is characterized by perihilar linear streaks on chest X-ray; neonatal respiratory distress syndrome is accompanied by ground-glass opacification of both lungs on CXR; and meconium aspiration syndrome is accompanied by patchy pulmonary infiltrates with possible pleural effusion on CXR.**
- **Finally, all of these three conditions may require oxygen therapy, depending on the severity.**
- This patient presents with an increased respiratory rate.
- His chest X-ray shows perihilar linear streaks consistent with fluid in the interlobar fissures.
- This description is consistent with transient tachypnea of the newborn (TTN).
- Diagnosis of TTN is further supported by the fact that this patient was born via cesarean delivery. Neonates born via cesarean delivery are unable to clear their alveolar fluid completely. Retention of this alveolar fluid is exactly what causes tachypnea in patients with this condition.

Pediatrics | Section 10: GI Disease - Hypertrophic Pyloric Stenosis, Intussusception & Malrotation with Volvulus

I. Hypertrophic Pyloric Stenosis: Definition
   A. Thickening and lengthening of gastric pylorus ~ 2 - 6 weeks after birth
   B. Most common cause of gastric outlet obstruction in infants
   C. More common in firstborn males

II. Hypertrophic Pyloric Stenosis: Etiology
   A. Not completely understood
   B. Associated with macrolide exposure before or shortly after birth

III. Hypertrophic Pyloric Stenosis: Clinical Presentation
   A. Palpable olive-shaped epigastric mass
   B. Visible peristaltic waves
   C. Projectile vomiting

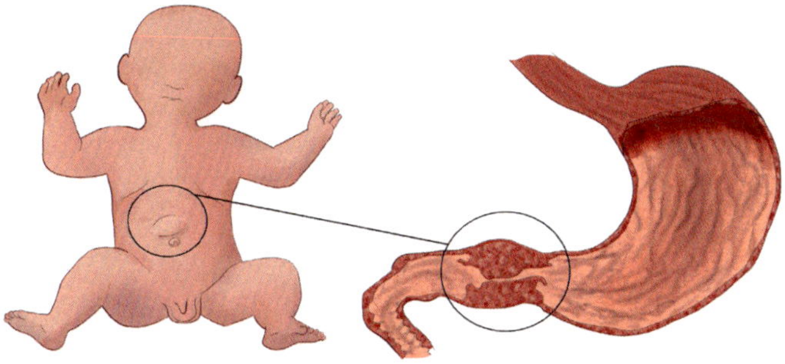

FIGURE 18.1.26 - Hypertrophic Pyloric Stenosis

IV. Hypertrophic Pyloric Stenosis: Diagnosis
   A. Hypokalemic hypochloremic metabolic alkalosis due to:
      1. Loss of gastric acid
      2. Volume contraction activating renin-angiotensin-aldosterone system
   B. Abdominal ultrasoun
      1. Thickened and lengthened pylorus
      2. Narrowed pyloric channel

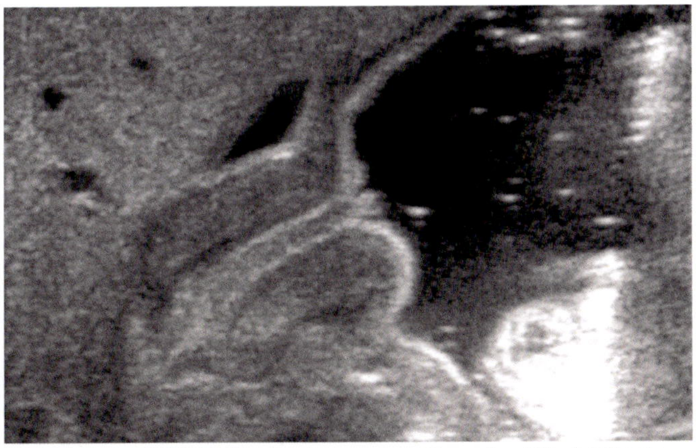

FIGURE 18.1.27 - Abdominal Ultrasound: Thickened Pyloric Walls and Narrowed Pyloric Channel in Hypertrophic Pyloric Stenosis

V. Hypertrophic Pyloric Stenosis: Management
   A. Volume resuscitation and electrolyte correction before surgery
   B. Surgical incision of pyloric muscles (pyloromyotomy)

VI. Intussusception: Definition
   A. Telescoping of proximal bowel segment into the distal bowel segment
   B. Most common at the ileocecal junction

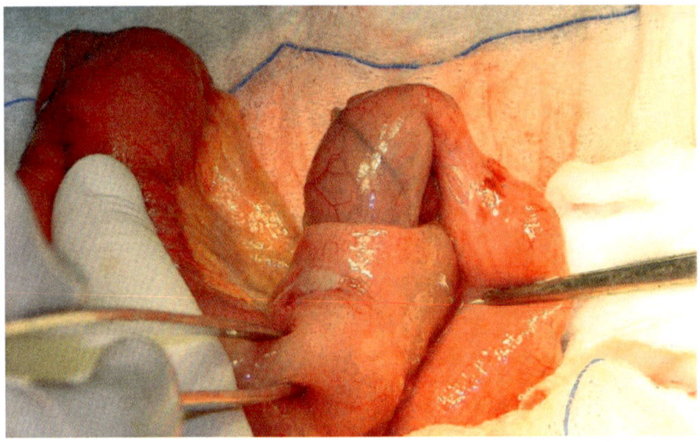

FIGURE 18.1.28 - Intussusception

VII. Intussusception: Etiology
   A. Most commonly idiopathic
   B. Due to lead point
      1. Meckel diverticulum (children)
      2. Intraluminal tumor (adults)
      3. Peyer patch hypertrophy due to:
         a) Henoch-Schonlein purpura
         b) Recent viral GI infection

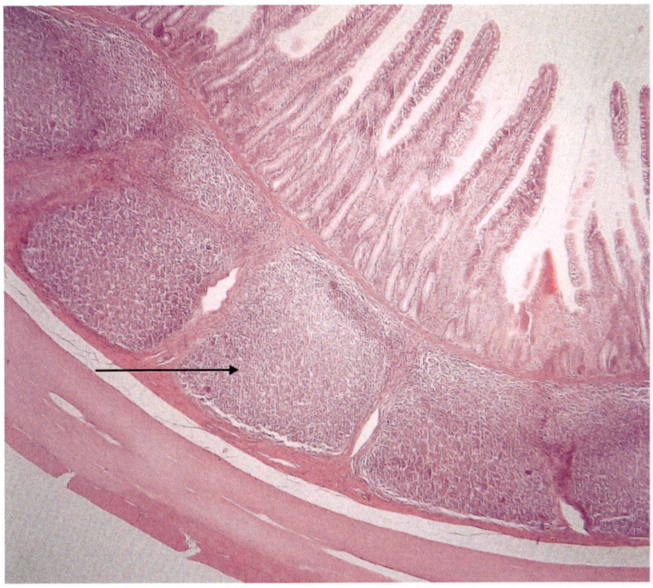

FIGURE 18.1.29 - Light Microscopy: Peyer Patches

VIII. Intussusception: Clinical Presentation
- A. Intermittent abdominal pain with "currant jelly" dark red stools due to ischemia and necrosis of proximal bowel segment
- B. Sausage-shaped mass in the right abdomen
- C. Drawing legs to chest relieves the pain (fetal position)

IX. Intussusception: Diagnosis
- A. Ultrasound or CT
  1. Target sign: concentric layers of telescoped proximal bowel

X. Intussusception: Management
- A. Water soluble contrast or air enema: diagnostic and therapeutic
- B. Laparotomy if enema is unsuccessful or there are signs of bowel perforation and necrosis
  1. Hypotension
  2. Lactic acidosis
  3. Rebound tenderness
  4. Abdominal rigidity

XI. Malrotation with Volvulus: Definition
- A. Malrotation
  1. Incomplete rotation of midgut around superior mesenteric artery during weeks 6 - 10 of gestation
- B. Volvulus
  1. Twisting of bowel around its mesentery

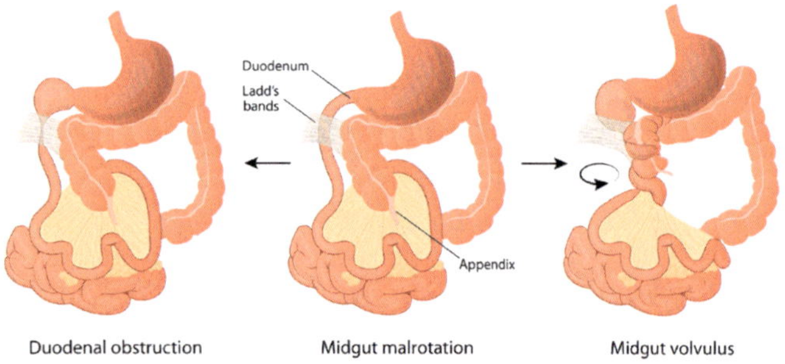

FIGURE 18.1.30 - Midgut Malrotation

XII. Malrotation with Volvulus: Etiology
- A. Malrotation: unknown
- B. Volvulus
  1. Malrotation (infants and children)
  2. Constipation (elderly)

XIII. Malrotation with Volvulus: Clinical Presentation
- A. Malrotation
  1. Mostly asymptomatic
  2. Constipation and bilious vomiting
- B. Volvulus
  1. Abdominal pain
  2. Obstipation (inability to pass stool and gas)
  3. Signs of peritonitis in case of bowel rupture (e.g. rigidity)

XIV. Malrotation with Volvulus: Diagnosis
- A. Malrotation
  1. Upper GI series with barium swallow: "corkscrew" bowel and right-sided ligament of Treitz
- B. Volvulus
  1. Abdominal X-ray: "coffee bean" sign directed to the left (midgut) or right (sigmoid) upper quadrant
  2. Midgut volvulus in children; sigmoid volvulus in elderly

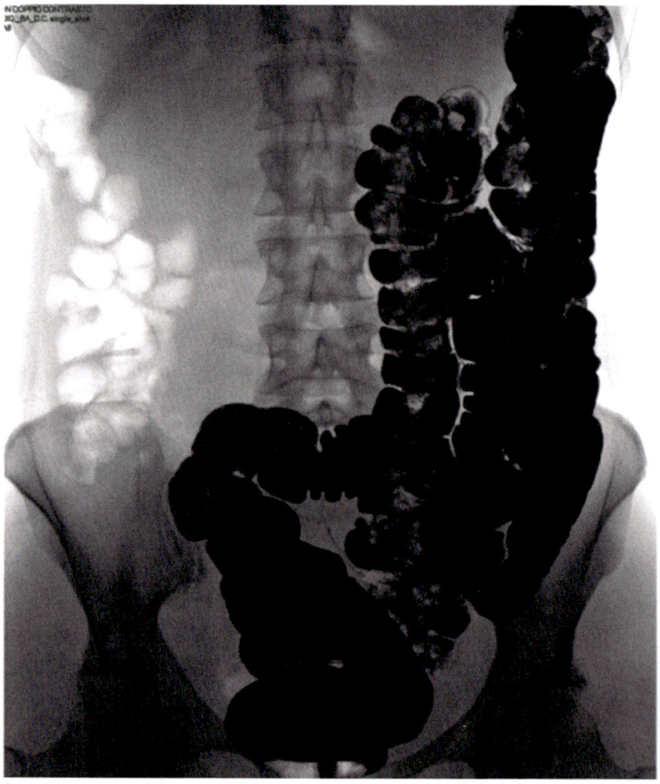

FIGURE 18.1.31 - Barium Enema: Intestinal Malrotation

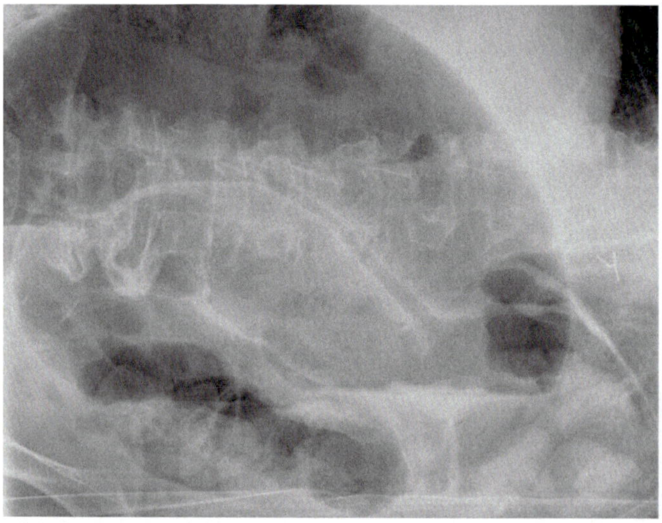

FIGURE 18.1.32 - X-ray of the Abdomen: "Coffee-Bean" Sign in Sigmoid Volvulus

XV. Malrotation with Volvulus: Management
  A. Malrotation
    1. Ladd procedure: surgical lysis of Ladd bands and bowel fixation in its normal location
  B. Volvulus
    1. Surgical detorsion

Condition	Etiology	Key Features
Hypertrophic pyloric stenosis	- More common in firstborn males - Associated with macrolide exposure of infant	- Palpable, olive-shaped epigastric mass - Visible peristaltic waves - Hypokalemic hypochloremic metabolic alkalosis - Medical treatment: correction of electrolyte imbalance and volume status before surgery - Surgical treatment: pyloromyotomy

Intussusception	- Telescoping of proximal bowel segment into distal bowel segment
	- Lead point:
	  - Meckel diverticulum (children)
	  - Intraluminal tumor (adults)
	  - Peyer patch hypertrophy (e.g. Henoch-Schonlein purpura, viral GI infection)
		- "Currant jelly" stools
		- "Target sign" on ultrasound/CT
		- Diagnosis and treatment: water soluble contrast or air enema
		- Laparotomy if enema is unsuccessful or there are signs of bowel perforation (e.g. rebound tenderness, rigidity)

Malrotation with volvulus	- Malrotation: incomplete rotation of midgut around SMA during 6-10 weeks of gestation - Volvulus: twisting of bowel around its mesentery	- Upper GI series with barium swallow: "corkscrew" bowel and right-sided ligament of Treitz in malrotation - Abdominal X-ray: coffee bean sign in volvulus - Midgut volvulus in children - Sigmoid volvulus in elderly - Treatment of malrotation: Ladd procedure (surgical lysis of Ladd bands) - Treatment of volvulus: surgical detorsion

TABLE 18.1.8 - Pediatric Gastrointestinal Diseases

REVIEW QUESTIONS

1. A 4-week-old boy is brought to his primary care physician because vomiting and weight loss for the past week. He is constantly hungry. The physical exam shows an olive-shaped epigastric mass, decreased skin turgor, and visible peristaltic waves. Laboratory findings are significant for hypokalemic hypochloremic metabolic alkalosis. What is the best initial treatment for this patient?
   - **The best initial treatment for this patient is correction of volume and electrolyte status.**
   - This patient presents with vomiting and weight loss for the past week.
   - The physical exam shows an olive-shaped epigastric mass, decreased skin turgor, and visible peristaltic waves.
   - These findings are consistent with the diagnosis of hypertrophic pyloric stenosis.
   - Laboratory findings are significant for hypokalemic hypochloremic metabolic alkalosis.
   - These electrolyte and acid-base abnormalities result from loss of gastric acid and the activation of the renin-angiotensin-aldosterone system by volume contraction.
   - The best initial treatment for hypertrophic pyloric stenosis is correction of volume and electrolyte status before pyloromyotomy.

REVIEW QUESTIONS

2. A 3-year-old girl is brought to her primary care physician because of abdominal pain and dark red stools for the past day. She draws her knees to her chest to relieve the pain. She had multiple episodes of watery diarrhea and vomiting before her current complaints. The physical exam shows a sausage-shaped mass in the right lower quadrant. What will most likely be found on the ultrasound of this patient?

    - **The ultrasound of this patient will most likely show the target sign, which represents the concentric layers of the telescoped proximal bowel.**
    - This patient presents with abdominal pain and dark red stools for the past day. She draws her knees to her chest to relieve the pain.
    - The physical exam shows a sausage-shaped mass in the right lower quadrant.
    - These findings are consistent with the diagnosis of intussusception.
    - She had multiple episodes of watery diarrhea and vomiting before her current complaints. This is consistent with viral gastroenteritis. Viral gastroenteritis likely induced hypertrophy of Peyer patches which acted as the lead point for intussusception.

3. A 3-year-old girl is brought to her primary care physician because of constipation and intermittent bilious vomiting for the past week. Upper GI series with barium swallow show irregular narrowings of the small bowel and a right-sided ligament of Treitz. What is the most likely pathophysiology of this patient's underlying condition?

    - **The most likely pathophysiology of this patient's underlying condition is incomplete rotation of the midgut around the superior mesenteric artery during 6 to 10 weeks of gestation.**
    - This patient presents with constipation and intermittent bilious vomiting.
    - Upper GI series with barium swallow show irregular narrowings of the small bowel and the right-sided ligament of Treitz.
    - These findings confirm the diagnosis of malrotation, which is caused by incomplete rotation of the midgut around the superior mesenteric artery during 6 to 10 weeks of gestation.

4. A 4-year-old boy is brought to the physician by his parents because of abdominal pain and dark red stools for the past day. He has never had such symptoms before. He had two episodes of watery diarrhea and vomiting before his current complaints. His vital signs are normal. The physical exam shows a child in severe distress drawing his knees to his chest to relieve the pain. There is no rebound tenderness or abdominal rigidity. An abdominal ultrasound shows concentric layers of bowel in the right lower quadrant. Which of the following is the best initial step in the management of this patient?

    A. IV ampicillin
    B. Polyethylene glycol
    C. Water soluble enema
    D. Laparotomy

    - **The correct answer is option C.**
    - This 4-year-old boy presents with abdominal pain and dark red stools, also known as "currant jelly stools", for the past day. The physical exam shows a child in severe distress drawing his knees to his chest to relieve the pain.
    - An abdominal ultrasound shows concentric layers of bowel in the right lower quadrant. This description is consistent with the "target sign."
    - All these clues suggest the diagnosis of intussusception.
    - The best initial step in the management of a patient with intussusception is water soluble enema, which is both diagnostic and therapeutic.
    - Option A, intravenous (IV) ampicillin, is incorrect because antibiotics are not indicated in intussusception unless the patient has signs of infection.
    - Option B, polyethylene glycol, is incorrect because it is an osmotic laxative. Laxatives are contraindicated in intussusception due to potential for bowel obstruction at the ileocecal junction.
    - Option D, laparotomy, is incorrect because it is used when the enema is unsuccessful or the patient has signs of bowel perforation and necrosis. This patient has a benign abdominal exam with no rebound tenderness or abdominal rigidity.

Pediatrics | Section 11: GI Disease - Meckel Diverticulum, Hirschsprung Disease & Necrotizing Enterocolitis

I. Meckel Diverticulum: Definition
   A. True congenital diverticulum in the terminal ileum
   B. Most common congenital GI tract anomaly
   C. May contain heterotopic gastric mucosa and/or pancreatic tissue

II. Meckel Diverticulum: Etiology
   A. Incomplete resorption of proximal vitelline (omphalomesenteric) duct

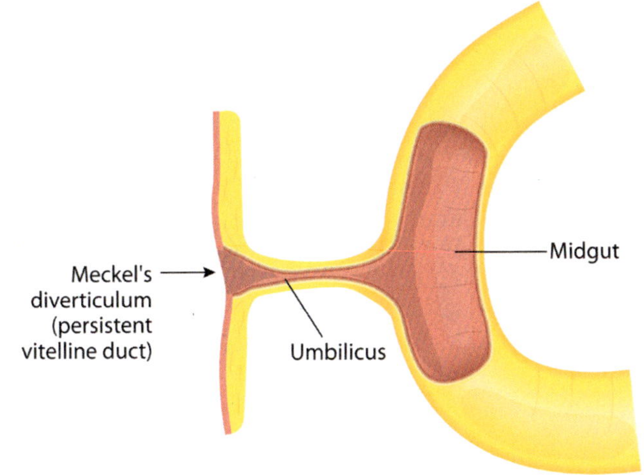

FIGURE 18.1.33 - Meckel's Diverticulum

III. Meckel Diverticulum: Clinical Presentation
   a. Most commonly asymptomatic
   A. Right lower quadrant pain
   B. Hematochezia or melena
   C. Intussusception

IV. Meckel Diverticulum: Diagnosis
   A. ^{99m}Tc-pertechnetate scan (Meckel scan)
      1. Signal from stomach and the terminal ileum

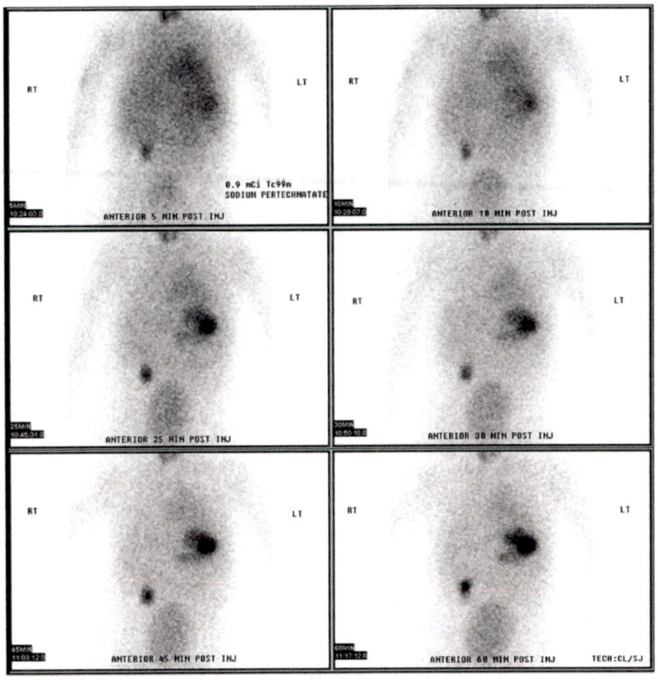

FIGURE 18.1.34 - Meckel Scan

V. Meckel Diverticulum: Management
   A. Observation if asymptomatic
   B. Surgical excision if symptomatic

VI. Hirschsprung Disease: Definition
   A. Absence of Auerbach and Meissner plexuses in the sigmoid colon and rectum

VII. Hirschsprung Disease: Etiology
   A. Congenital
      1. Failure of neural crest cell migration to the distal colon
      2. Loss of function mutation in *RET* gene
      3. Associated with Down syndrome
   B. Acquired
      1. Chagas disease by *Trypanosoma cruzi*

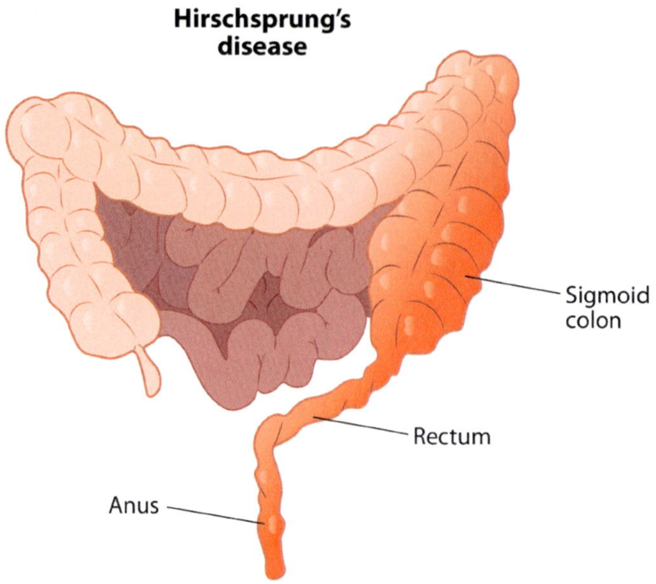

FIGURE 18.1.35 - Hirschsprung Disease

VIII. Hirschsprung Disease: Clinical Presentation
  A. Bilious vomiting
  B. Abdominal distension
  C. Delayed passage of meconium
  D. Chronic constipation

IX. Hirschsprung Disease: Diagnosis
  A. Squirt sign
    1. Explosive expulsion of feces on digital rectal exam
  B. Rectal manometry
    1. Increased pressure in rectum and sigmoid colon
  C. Rectal suction biopsy
    1. Absence of Auerbach and Meissner's plexus in colonic wall

X. Hirschsprung Disease: Management
  A. Surgical resection of aganglionic segment

XI. Necrotizing Enterocolitis: Definition
  A. Intestinal inflammation and necrosis in infants
  B. Most commonly affects the terminal ileum and cecum

XII. Necrotizing Enterocolitis: Etiology
  A. Invasion of GI mucosa by gas-producing bacteria → intestinal necrosis

XIII. Necrotizing Enterocolitis: Risk Factors
  A. Very low birth weight (< 1.5 kg)
  B. Prematurity
  C. Enteral feeding

XIV. Necrotizing Enterocolitis: Clinical Presentation
  A. Nonspecific signs
    1. Apnea, lethargy, fussiness
    2. Septic shock (hypotension, tachycardia, fever)
  B. Gastrointestinal signs
    1. Feeding intolerance and bilious emesis
    2. Abdominal distension and erythema
    3. Hematochezia

XV. Necrotizing Enterocolitis: Complications
  A. Disseminated intravascular coagulation
  B. Post-surgical complications
    1. Strictures
    2. Short-bowel syndrome

XVI. Necrotizing Enterocolitis: Diagnosis
  A. Abdominal X-ray
    1. Pneumatosis intestinalis (air in bowel wall)
    2. Pneumoperitoneum (bowel rupture)
  B. Blood cultures

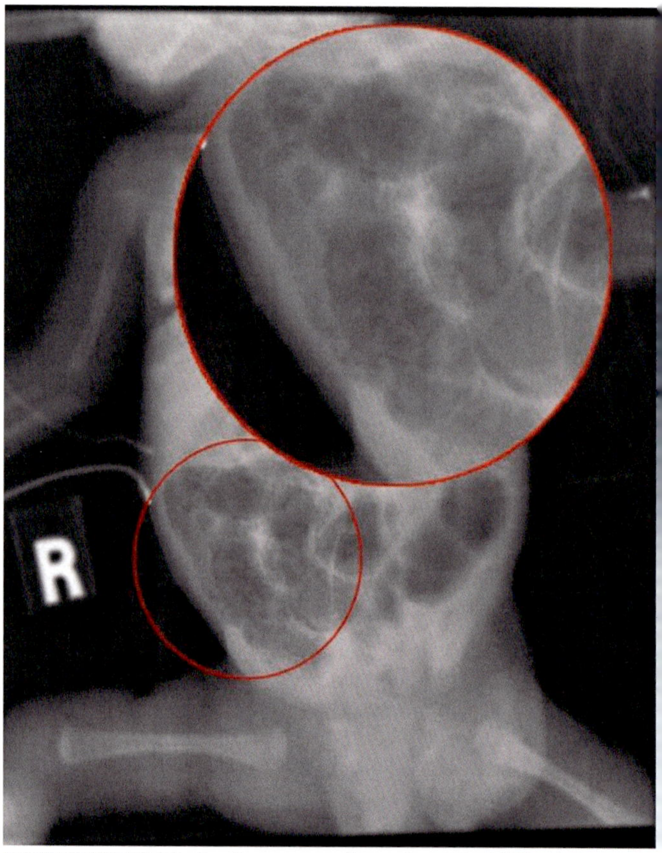

FIGURE 18.1.36 - Abdominal X-ray: Pneumatosis Intestinalis in Necrotizing Enterocolitis

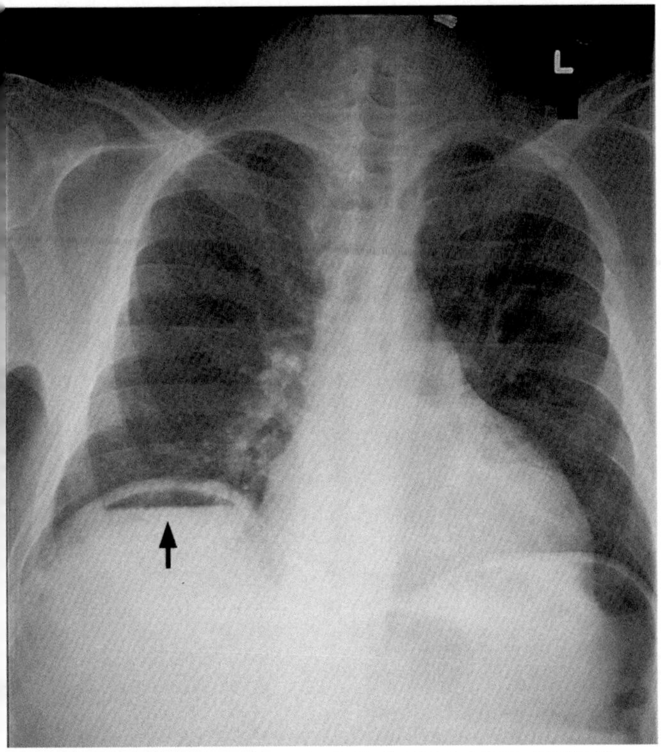

FIGURE 18.1.37 - Chest X-ray: Pneumoperitoneum

XVII. Necrotizing Enterocolitis: Management
- A. Nil per os (NPO) regimen
- B. Nasogastric decompression
- C. IV fluids followed by empiric antibiotics
- D. Indications for surgery
    1. Pneumoperitoneum (bowel perforation)
    2. Clinical deterioration despite optimal medical management (bowel necrosis)

Condition	Etiology	Key Features
Meckel diverticulum	- Most common congenital GI tract anomaly - Remnant of vitelline duct	- Diagnosed by 99mTc-pertechnetate (Meckel) scan - May contain heterotopic gastric and/or pancreatic tissue - Asymptomatic: observation - Symptomatic: surgical excision
Hirschsprung disease	- Absence of Auerbach and Meissner's plexus in sigmoid colon and rectum - Congenital: failure of neural crest cell migration due to loss of function mutation in *RET* gene - Acquired: Chagas disease by *Trypanosoma cruzi*	- Congenital Hirschsprung disease associated with Down syndrome - Positive squirt sign and increased rectal pressure - Diagnosed with rectal suction biopsy - Surgical excision of aganglionic segment
Necrotizing enterocolitis	- Intestinal inflammation and necrosis due to penetration of gas-producing bacteria in GI wall	- Associated with very low birth weight (< 1.5 kg), prematurity, enteral feeding - Pneumatosis intestinalis (air in bowel wall) on X-ray - Treatment: NPO regimen, nasogastric decompression, IV fluids, and empiric antibiotics - Indications for surgery: - Pneumoperitoneum, clinical deterioration despite medical management

TABLE 18.1.9 - Pediatric Gastrointestinal Diseases

REVIEW QUESTIONS

?

1. A 2-year-old boy is brought to the physician due to bloody stools for the past 2 days. He also has right lower quadrant pain. Right lower quadrant ultrasound shows a protruding mass near the ileocecal valve. ^{99m}Tc-pertechnetate scan reveals increased signal from the terminal ileum. What is the most likely pathophysiology of this patient's current condition?

- **The most likely pathophysiology of this patient's current condition is incomplete resorption of the proximal vitelline duct during fetal period.**
- This patient presents with bloody stools and right lower quadrant pain.
- The right lower quadrant ultrasound shows a protruding mass near the ileocecal valve.
- 99mTc-pertechnetate scan reveals an increased signal from the terminal ileum.
- These findings are consistent with the diagnosis of a Meckel diverticulum.
- Meckel diverticulum is caused by incomplete resorption of the proximal vitelline duct during the fetal period.

2. A 2-year-old girl with Down syndrome presents with chronic constipation and intermittent bilious vomiting. The physician observes an explosive expulsion of feces on digital rectal exam. Rectal tone is increased on rectal manometry. Abdominal X-ray reveals an enlarged descending colon with a narrow sigmoid colon and rectum. Which test can definitively diagnose this patient's condition?

- **The test that can definitively diagnose this patient's condition is a rectal suction biopsy.**
- This patient presents with chronic constipation and intermittent bilious vomiting.
- He has a history of Down syndrome.
- The physician observes an explosive expulsion of feces on the digital rectal exam.
- Rectal tone is increased on the rectal manometry.
- Abdominal X-ray shows an enlarged descending colon with a narrow sigmoid colon and rectum.
- All these findings suggest the diagnosis of Hirschsprung disease.
- Hirschsprung disease can be definitively diagnosed with rectal suction biopsy.

1. A 3-week-old boy is brought to the primary care physician because of fussiness and poor feeding for the last 3 days. He was born at 34 weeks of gestation with a birth weight of 1 kg. His vital signs include temperature of 102.2° F (39° C), blood pressure of 60/35 mmHg, heart rate of 175 beats/min, and respiratory rate of 62 breaths/min. The physical exam shows diffuse abdominal tenderness with no rigidity. Abdominal X-ray shows gas in the bowel wall but no air in the peritoneal cavity. He is placed on NPO regimen, and he undergoes nasogastric decompression. Which of the following is the best next step in the management of this patient?
   A. IV fluids
   B. IV antibiotics
   C. Blood culture
   D. Surgery

- **The correct answer is option A.**
- This patient presents with nonspecific symptoms of fussiness and poor feeding.
- He was born at 34 weeks of gestation with a birth weight of 1 kg. Therefore, he is premature with a very low birth weight.
- His vital signs show fever, hypotension, tachycardia, and tachypnea.
- Abdominal X-ray shows gas in the bowel wall but no air in the peritoneal cavity.
- These findings are consistent with the diagnosis of necrotizing enterocolitis.
- He is placed on NPO regimen, and he undergoes nasogastric decompression.
- The best next step in the management of this patient is intravenous fluids to increase blood pressure to the normal range.
- Option B is incorrect because antibiotics are administered after a blood culture is obtained. IV fluids are prioritized to support this patient hemodynamically.
- Option C is incorrect because blood culture is usually done after IV fluids are initiated.
- Option D is incorrect because surgery is performed when the patient has pneumoperitoneum or is deteriorating despite medical management. Therefore, one should first try medical management.

Pediatrics | Section 12: Urology - Cryptorchidism, Vesicoureteral Reflux & Posterior Urethral Valves

I. Cryptorchidism
   A. Most common congenital urogenital tract anomaly where one or both testicles fail to descend fully into the scrotum
   B. Risk factors: prematurity, low birth weight, DES exposure in utero, small for gestational age
   C. Clinical features: failure to palpate the testicle in the scrotum, hypoplastic scrotum, ↓ rugation of the scrotum; inguinal fullness
   D. Multiple locations (e.g. abdominal, inguinal)
   E. Diagnosis: mostly clinical
      1. Lab: ↓ testosterone (if bilateral), normal testosterone (if unilateral)
   F. Management
      1. Cryptorchidism usually resolve spontaneously by age 4-6 months
      2. If not, orchidopexy should be performed before age of 1
   G. Complications: infertility/subfertility, testicular cancer, testicular torsion, inguinal hernia

II. Vesicoureteral Reflux: General Information
   A. Retrograde flow of urine from the bladder and into the ureters
   B. Girls > boys (2:1)

III. Vesicoureteral Reflux: Etiology
   A. Primary (more common): short intramural part of the ureter
   B. Secondary: bladder outlet obstruction (e.g. posterior urethral valves, urethral meatal stenosis, neurogenic bladder), congenital ureteral anomalies, iatrogenic (post surgery)

IV. Vesicoureteral Reflux: Clinical Features
   A. Prenatally detected hydronephrosis/oligohydramnios
   B. Asymptomatic
   C. Recurrent UTI: fever, irritability (neonates); urgency, frequency, dysuria (older children); flank/abdominal pain
   D. Complications
      1. Nephropathy (interstitial nephritis), hypertension, kidney failure, renal scarring, urosepsis

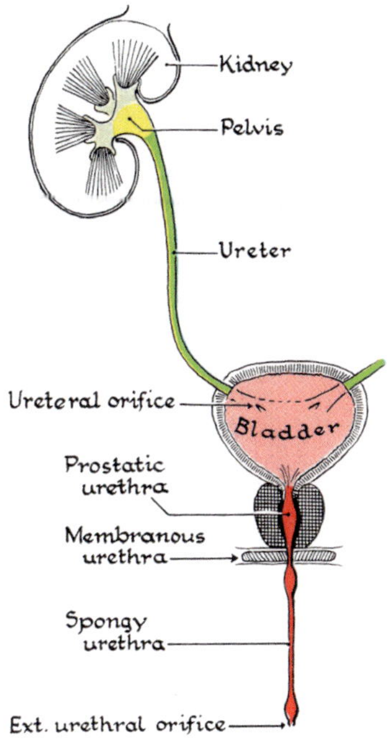

Grant, John Charles Boileau, Public domain, via Wikimedia Commons

FIGURE 18.1.39 - The Urinary System

V. Vesicoureteral Reflux: Diagnosis
   A. Laboratory examination
      1. Urinalysis and urine culture
      2. Renal function tests: to look for evidence of reflux nephropathy
         a) Serial creatinine, urea
      3. CBC: anemia, leukocytosis
   B. Ultrasound
      1. Antenatal ultrasound may show evidence of hydronephrosis
      2. Postnatally in all patients with febrile UTI: hydronephrosis
      3. Follow-up
   C. Contrast voiding cystourethrogram (VCUG): reflux of urine from the bladder into the ureters during micturition
      1. Classifies severity: grades I-V

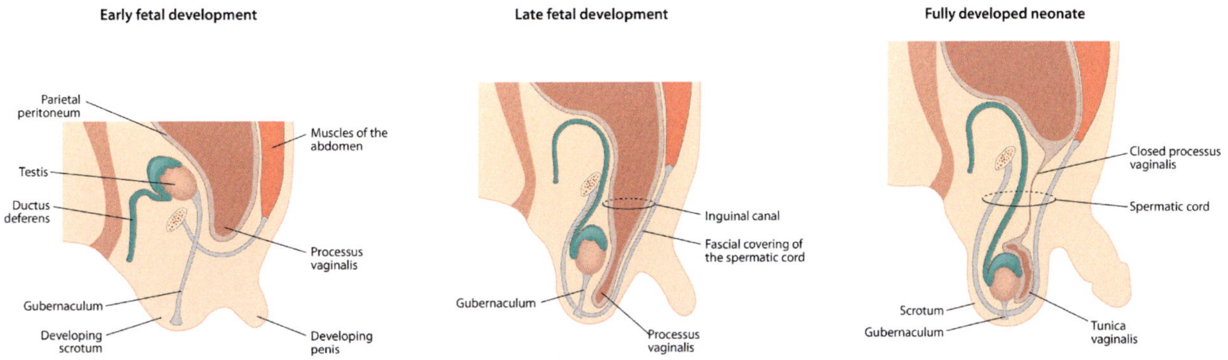

FIGURE 18.1.38 - Pathway of Normal Descent of the Testicle

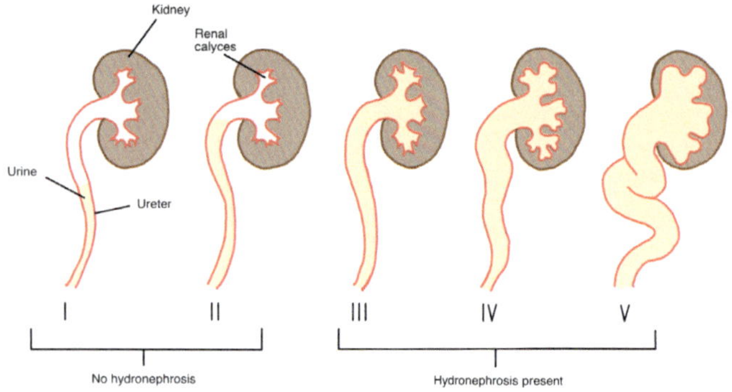

FIGURE 18.1.40 - Grades of Vesicoureteral Reflux

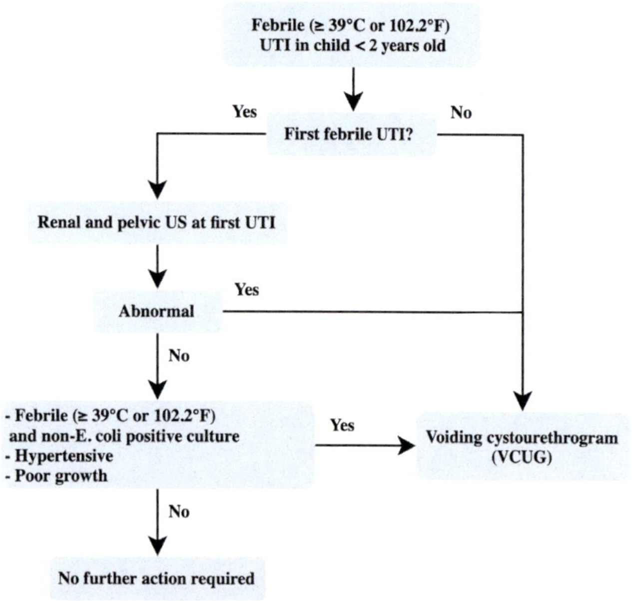

FIGURE 18.1.41 - Management of Febrile UTI in Child < 2 Years of Age

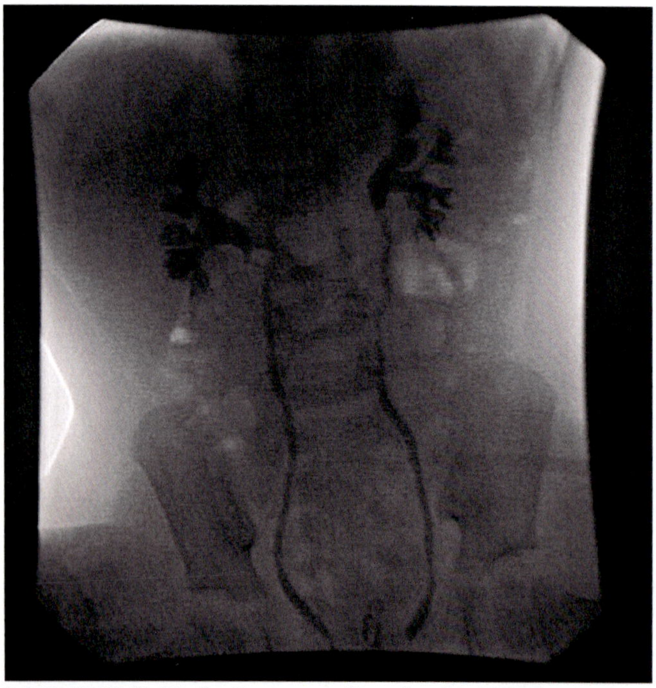

FIGURE 18.1.42 - Voiding Cystourethrogram: Bilateral Vesicoureteral Reflux

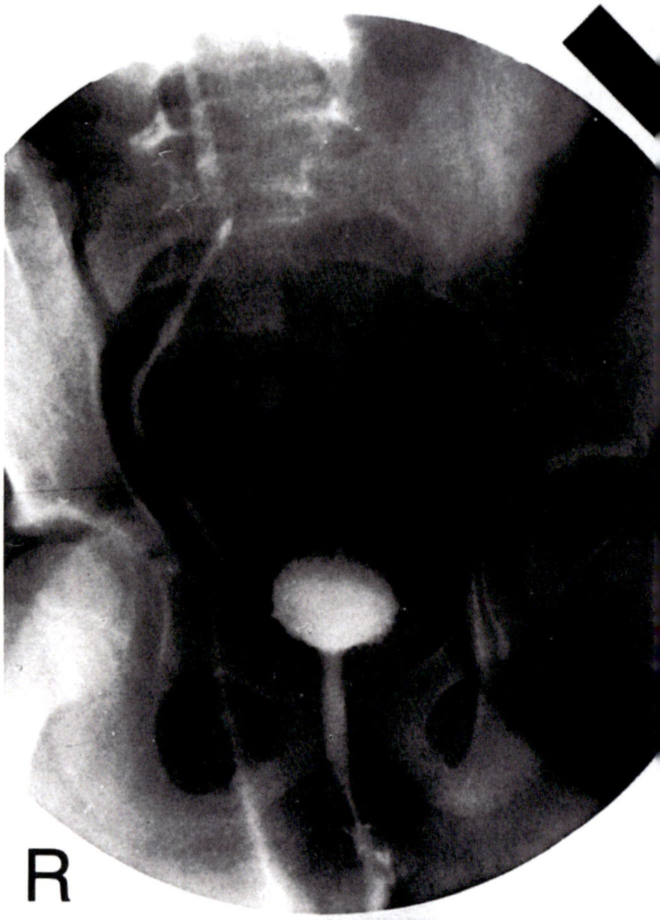

FIGURE 18.1.43 - Voiding Cystourethrogram: Unilateral Vesicoureteral Reflux

VI. Vesicoureteral Reflux: Management
   A. Initial management: treat infection
   B. Patients with low risk of pyelonephritis and renal scarring (children < 5 years with grades 1 - 3)
      1. Long-term prophylactic antibiotics; monitor closely with urinalysis and renal imaging
   C. Patients with high risk (grades 4 - 5, bilateral VUR, refractory disease despite treatment)
      1. Surgery: ureteral transplantation (high success rate)
   D. Renal scintigraphy with dimercaptosuccinic acid: for long-term evaluation of renal scarring

VII. Posterior Urethral Valves
   A. Congenital anomaly in boys where membranous folds obstruct urinary flow in the distal prostatic urethra
   B. This causes the urine to back up into the bladder and ureters → progressive bladder dilation, ureteral dilation → hydronephrosis
   C. Most common cause of urinary bladder obstruction in newborn males

VIII. Posterior Urethral Valves: Clinical Features
   A. Respiratory distress: Potter's sequence (flat facies, pulmonary hypoplasia, and limb deformities)
   B. Abdominal distension (distension of the bladder)
   C. Voiding problems: straining, poor urinary stream
   D. VUR, urinary tract infections, urosepsis, renal failure
   E. Failure to thrive

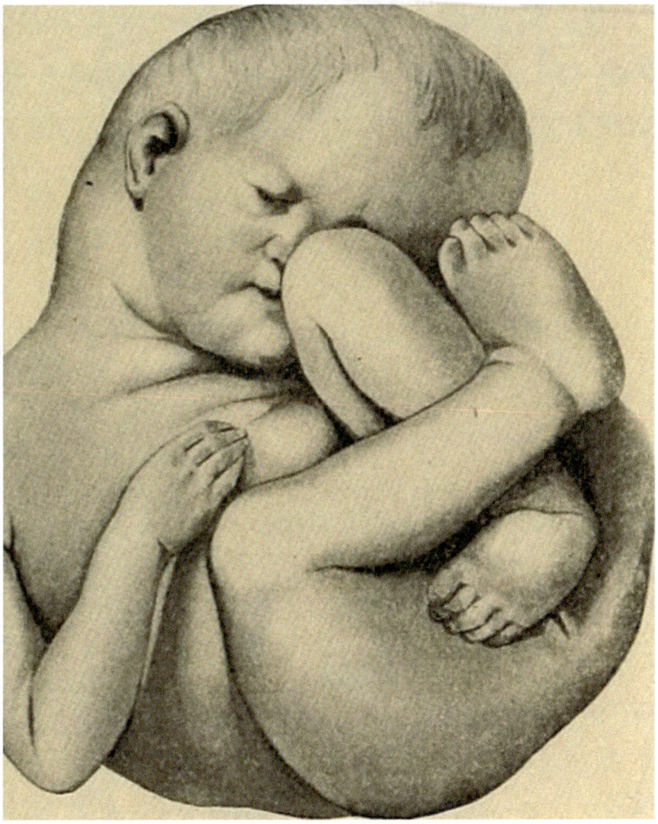

FIGURE 18.1.44 - Potter Sequence

IX. Posterior Urethral Valves: Diagnosis and Management
   A. Diagnosis
      1. Voiding cystourethrogram (method of choice): dilation of prostatic urethra
      2. Ultrasound: thick, dilated bladder; bilateral hydronephrosis
   B. Management
      1. Valve ablation: 1st line

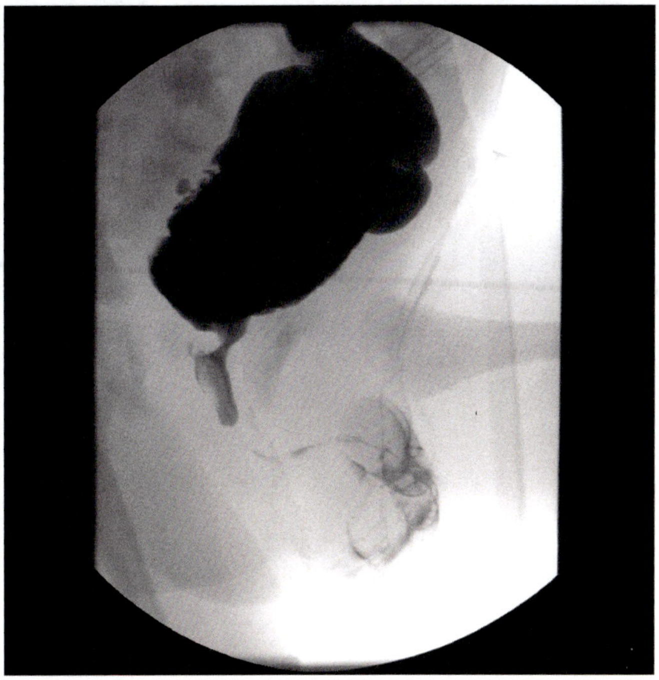

FIGURE 18.1.45 - Posterior Urethral Valve

REVIEW QUESTIONS

1. A 6-month-old boy is brought to the primary care physician for a well-child examination. He is at the 60th percentile for length and 70th percentile for weight. Physical examination shows only one testicle is palpated in the scrotum, but the examination is otherwise normal. What is the recommended treatment for this patient's condition?
   - **The recommended treatment for this patient's condition is orchidopexy.**
   - This 6-month-old boy has only one testicle palpated in the scrotum, which is consistent with cryptorchidism.
   - Since he's 6 months old, orchidopexy is the recommended treatment because spontaneous descent of the testes is very unlikely after this age. Orchidopexy will prevent complications such as infertility and testicular cancer and should be performed before the age of 1 year.

REVIEW QUESTIONS

2. A 15-month-old girl is brought to the primary care physician due to irritability and fever for the past 2 days. Her mother says she cried every time she passed urine for the past 2 days. She was treated for a urinary tract infection 4 months ago, but is otherwise healthy. A renal ultrasound shows hydronephrosis of the right kidney. What is the best next step in management of this patient?

    - **The best next step in management of this patient is a voiding cystourethrography.**
    - This 15-month-old girl is presenting with irritability, fever, and crying while passing urine, which are signs and symptoms of an upper urinary tract infection.
    - She has been treated for a previous UTI , so this is a recurrent infection.
    - Renal ultrasound shows hydronephrosis.
    - All of these features suggest vesicoureteral reflux as the most likely diagnosis.
    - Therefore, a voiding cystourethrography is the best next step. It will measure the reflux of urine from the bladder into the ureters during micturition and will classify the severity of the reflux into grades from I-V.

3. A 10-day-old newborn boy is brought to the primary care physician because of high fever, irritability, and lack of feeding for 2 days. The pregnancy was complicated with oligohydramnios. On physical exam, his abdomen appears distended and his urine stream is weak. What is the method of choice to confirm the diagnosis of this patient?

    - **The method of choice to confirm the diagnosis of this patient is voiding cystourethrogram.**
    - This 10-day-old newborn boy is presenting with high fever, irritability, lack of feeding, and signs of urinary tract infection.
    - Oligohydramnios, distended abdomen, and weak urinary stream are all characteristic of posterior urethral valves.
    - Posterior urethral valves is the most common cause of urinary tract obstruction in newborn males. On ultrasound, a thick, dilated bladder and bilateral hydronephrosis are characteristic.
    - However, the method of choice for diagnosing posterior urethral valves is voiding cystourethrogram, which shows dilation of the prostatic urethra.

4. A newborn boy is being evaluated in the delivery room for weak cry, irregular breathing, and respiratory distress. His pulse oximetry shows an oxygen saturation of 76%. The pregnancy was complicated by oligohydramnios. Physical examination shows facial dysmorphisms and limb deformities. He has low-set ears, flat nose, and a small jaw. Breath sounds are decreased bilaterally. Ultrasound examination shows dilation of the ureters bilaterally as well as dilation of the bladder. Which of the following is the next step to confirm the diagnosis of the patient?

    A. Chest X-ray
    B. Nasogastric tube insertion
    C. Voiding cystourethrogram
    D. Karyotyping

    - **The correct answer is option C.**
    - This newborn male has irregular breathing, is in respiratory distress due to pulmonary hypoplasia, and has limb deformities, and facial abnormalities due to oligohydramnios.
    - This is consistent with Potter's sequence.
    - Ultrasound examination shows dilation of the ureters bilaterally as well as dilation of the bladder characteristic of posterior urethral valves.
    - Therefore, the next step to confirm the diagnosis is ordering voiding cystourethrogram.
    - Option A is incorrect because chest X-ray will reveal pulmonary hypoplasia and will explain the symptoms of respiratory distress. However, it will not reveal the underlying cause.
    - Option B is incorrect because nasogastric tube insertion is helpful to diagnose patients with esophageal atresia, commonly associated with tracheoesophageal fistula. However, tracheoesophageal fistula is associated with polyhydramnios, not oligohydramnios during pregnancy.
    - Option D is incorrect because karyotyping will confirm chromosomal abnormalities which are associated with facial and limb abnormalities, but the combination of these features along with the bladder and bilateral ureteral dilation is highly characteristic of urinary tract obstruction due to posterior urethral valves.

Pediatrics | Section 13: Urology - Penile Conditions

I. Epispadias
   A. Rare embryonic urogenital malformation where the urethra opens on the dorsal penis
   B. Commonly associated with bladder exstrophy
   C. Clinical diagnosis: dorsally located urethral opening, short phallus, dorsal penile curvature, urinary incontinence
   D. Complications: infertility, erectile dysfunction
   E. Management: surgical closure, urethroplasty

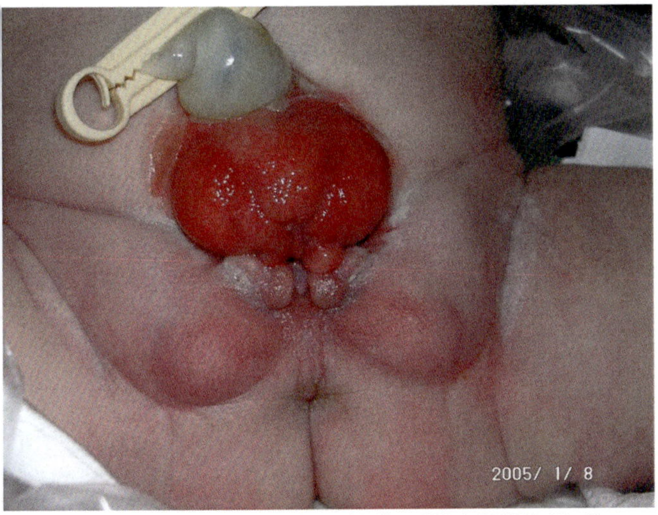

FIGURE 18.1.46 - Bladder Exstrophy

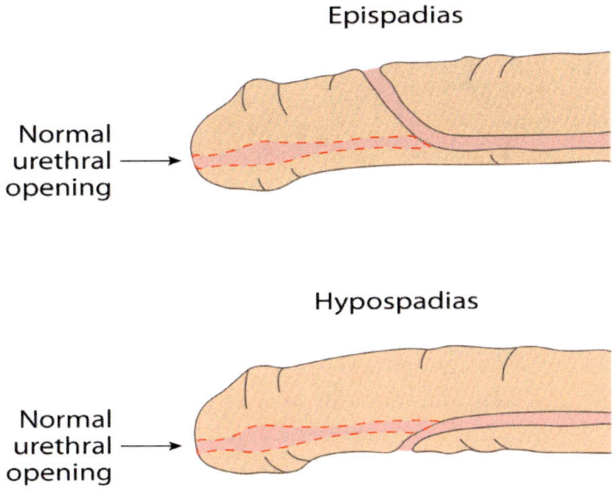

FIGURE 18.1.47 - Epispadias

II. Hypospadias
   A. Common embryonic urogenital malformation where urethra abnormally opens on the ventral penis due to failure of urethral folds to close
   B. Associated with syndromes (e.g. WAGR, Denys-Drash), ↓ androgen sensitivity, genetic disorders of sex development
   C. Clinical diagnosis: dorsal hood, ventrally located urethral opening, ventral penile curvature
   D. Circumcision is contraindicated: skin flap can be used in reconstruction
   E. Management
      1. Reconstruction surgery: urethroplasty, correction of the curvature if present

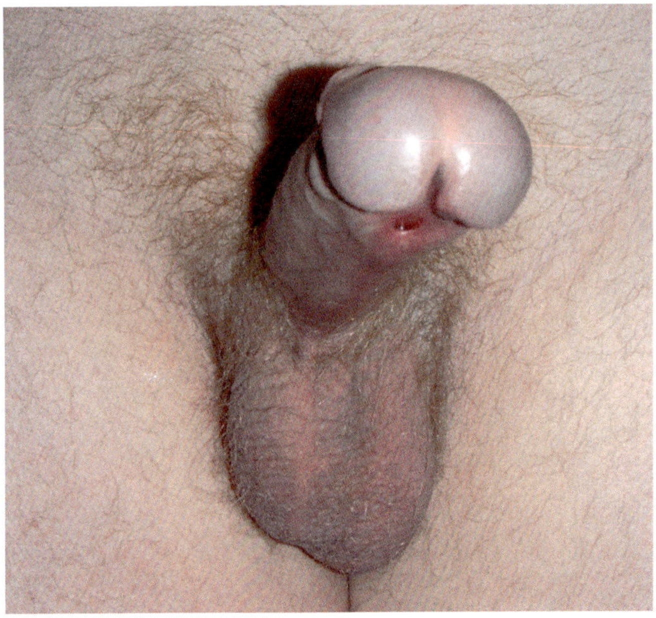

FIGURE 18.1.48 - Hypospadias

III. Phimosis
   A. Inability to completely retract the skin over the glans penis due to tight foreskin
      1. Physiologic: in uncircumcised newborns, resolves at age 6 - 7 years
      2. Pathologic: occurs as a result of inflammation and scarring
   B. Clinical diagnosis: inability to completely retract the foreskin, painful erection, dysuria, ballooning of the foreskin during urination
   C. Complications: tearing and bleeding, paraphimosis
   D. Management: depends on the extent and severity of the phimosis
      1. Daily gentle retraction and stretching
      2. Topical corticosteroid cream
      3. Circumcision (definitive treatment and the treatment of choice)

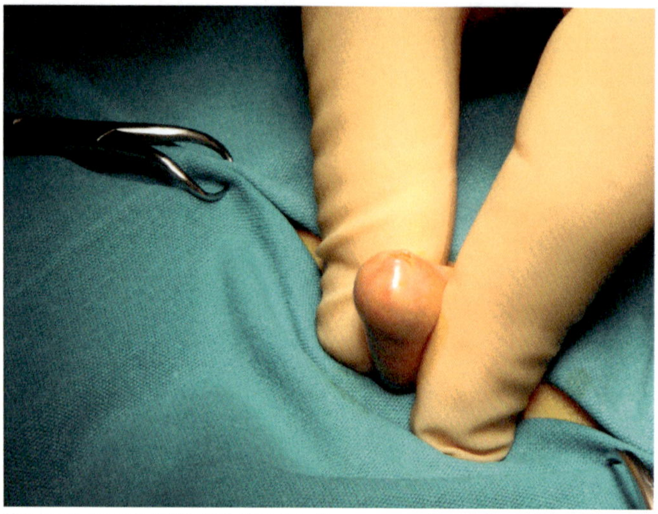

FIGURE 18.1.49 - Phimosis (Before Surgical Treatment)

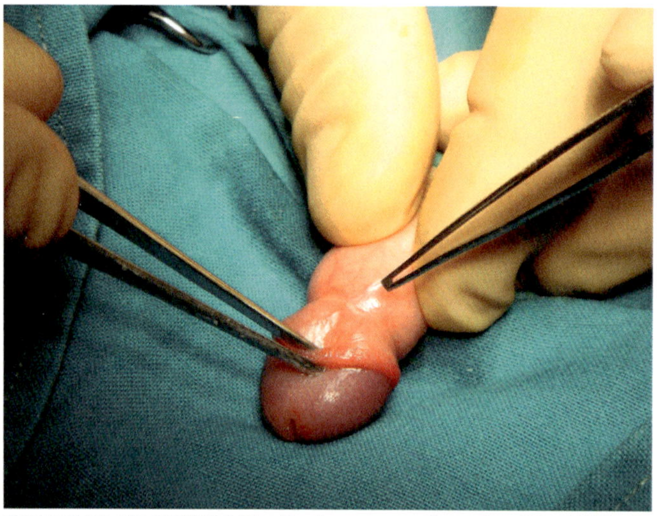

FIGURE 18.1.50 - After Surgical Treatment of Phimosis

IV. Paraphimosis
   A. A condition affecting uncircumcised males where the retracted foreskin cannot be pulled over the glans penis to its original position
   B. Etiology: complication of phimosis, iatrogenic (after retracting the foreskin for cleaning, for placing a urinary catheter)
   C. A medical emergency: foreskin is trapped → strangulation of the glans penis → vascular compromise → edema and possibly necrosis
   D. Clinical diagnosis: foreskin cannot be pulled to its original position, edematous foreskin, painful glans penis
   E. Management
      1. Manual reduction: for mild, uncomplicated cases
      2. Surgical treatment
         a) Incising the constricting band
         b) Circumcision (definitive treatment and the treatment of choice)

REVIEW QUESTIONS

1. A 2-day-old newborn boy presents with a urethral opening on the dorsal aspect of the penis. What other associated genitourinary abnormality is likely present in this patient?
   - **Bladder exstrophy is a congenital deformity that is often associated with epispadias.**
   - This 2-day-old newborn boy is presenting with epispadias suggested by the urethral opening on the dorsal aspect of the penis.

2. A three week old boy is brought to the emergency deparatment by his parents because of swelling of his penis. The patient was delivered vaginally with no complications, and his parents elected not to have him circumcised at the time of birth. Upon closer inspection of the newborn, it is noticed that his glans penis is swollen and the foreskin cannot be pulled back over it. The parents state they noticed it this morning and immediately rushed him to the office. What is the best treatment for this newborn's condition?

   A. Topical Corticosteroids
   B. Gentle Stretching
   C. Circumcision
   D. Urological Surgery

   - **The correct answer is option C.**
   - This three week old male is noticed to have swelling of his penis.
   - He is not circumcised.
   - The glans is swollen and the foreskin is stuck in the retracted position.
   - This is a condition known as paraphimosis, and it presents as an emergency due to possible strangulation of the glans penis.
   - The best and definitive treatment is circumcision.
   - Options A and B are incorrect because topical corticosteroids and gentle stretching are initial treatment options for phimosis, where the foreskin is stuck over the glans penis and unable to retract.
   - Option D is incorrect because circumcision is the definitive treatment for this patient's condition. Urological surgery is unnecessary, and would instead be used in the management of epispadias or hypospadias.

Pediatrics | Section 14: Congenital B Cell Immunodeficiencies

I. X-Linked Agammaglobulinemia: Definition
   A. Congenital immunodeficiency disorder characterized by absence of mature B cells
   B. Also known as Bruton agammaglobulinemia

II. X-Linked Agammaglobulinemia: Pathophysiology
   A. X-linked recessive defect in Bruton tyrosine kinase (BTK) leads to:
      1. Impaired B-cell maturation
      2. Decreased production of immunoglobulins
   B. Immunodeficiency manifests around 3 - 6 months of age
      1. Maternal antibodies confer protection until 3 - 6 months of age

III. X-Linked Agammaglobulinemia: Risk Factors
   A. Male sex

IV. X-Linked Agammaglobulinemia: Clinical Features
   A. Recurrent sinopulmonary infections (e.g. otitis media, pneumonia)
      1. Common culprits are encapsulated bacteria (e.g. *S. pneumoniae*)
   B. Recurrent gastrointestinal infections (e.g. *Giardia*, *Salmonella*)
   C. Scant or absent lymphoid tissue (e.g. tonsils, lymph nodes)

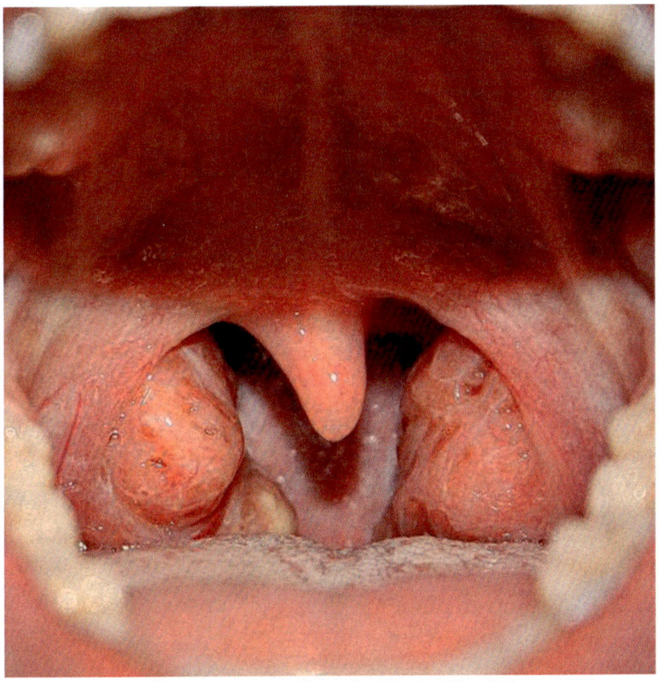

FIGURE 18.1.51 - The Uvula and Tonsils

V. X-linked Agammaglobulinemia: Diagnosis
   A. Quantitative measurement of immunoglobulins
      1. Decreased levels of all immunoglobulins
   B. Flow cytometry of peripheral blood smear
      1. Nearly absent $CD19^+$ B-cells
      2. Normal/high T-cell count
   C. Genetic testing confirms diagnosis

VI. X-Linked Agammaglobulinemia: Management
   A. Lifelong immunoglobulin replacement therapy
   B. Prophylactic antibiotics
   C. Vaccines do not produce an immunologic response
      1. Live vaccines are contraindicated

VII. Common Variable Immunodeficiency: Definition
   A. Congenital immunodeficiency disorder characterized by failure of B-cell differentiation

VIII. Common Variable Immunodeficiency: Pathophysiology
   A. Mature B-cells fail to differentiate into plasma cells
      1. Impaired production of all immunoglobulins

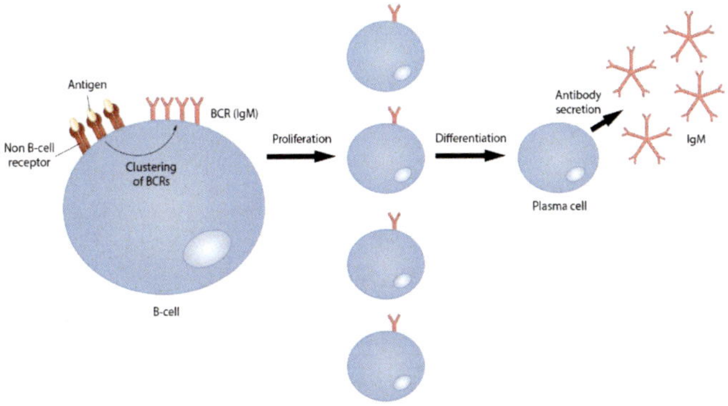

FIGURE 18.1.52 - Steps of Antibody Production

IX. Common Variable Immunodeficiency: Risk Factors
   A. Unknown

X. Common Variable Immunodeficiency: Clinical Features
   A. Presents during puberty or early adulthood
   B. Recurrent sinopulmonary infections (e.g. otitis media, pneumonia)
   C. Recurrent gastrointestinal infections (e.g. *Giardia*, *Salmonella*)
   D. Chronic lung disease (e.g. asthma, bronchiectasis)
   E. Chronic gastrointestinal tract disease (e.g. diarrhea, failure to thrive)
   F. Autoimmune manifestations (e.g. thyroid disease, arthritis)
   G. Increased risk for malignancy (e.g. lymphoma)

XI. Common Variable Immunodeficiency: Diagnosis
- A. Quantitative measurement of immunoglobulins
    1. Markedly decreased levels of IgG
    2. Decreased levels of other immunoglobulins (e.g. IgA, IgM)
- B. Normal B-cell and T-cell count
- C. Decreased plasma cell count

XII. Common Variable Immunodeficiency: Management
- A. Lifelong immunoglobulin replacement therapy
- B. Vaccines do not produce an immunologic response

XIII. Selective IgA Deficiency: Definition
- A. Congenital deficiency of IgA
- B. Most common primary immunodeficiency

XIV. Selective IgA Deficiency: Pathophysiology
- A. Plasma cells unable to produce IgA
- B. B-cell and T-cell function is normal

XV. Selective IgA Deficiency: Risk Factors
- A. Caucasians
- B. Family history

XVI. Selective IgA Deficiency: Clinical Features
- A. Asymptomatic
- B. Recurrent sinopulmonary and gastrointestinal infections
    1. Chronic giardiasis is common
- C. Association with autoimmune diseases (e.g. celiac disease)
- D. Association with atopic diseases (e.g. asthma, eczema)
- E. Increased risk of anaphylactic reaction to blood transfusions
    1. Patients with IgA deficiency may develop antibodies against IgA

XVII. Selective IgA Deficiency: Diagnosis
- A. Quantitative measurement of immunoglobulins
    1. Isolated deficiency of serum IgA
    2. Normal levels of other immunoglobulins (e.g. IgG, IgM)
- B. Normal B-cell and T-cell count

XVIII. Selective IgA Deficiency: Management
- A. Supportive care (e.g. treatment of recurrent infections)
- B. Medical alert bracelet to alert care teams about a possible blood transfusion reaction
- C. "Wash" packed red blood cells (pRBCs) prior to transfusion
    1. "Washing" means removing plasma from pRBCs

Immunodeficiency	Pathophysiology	Key Features	Diagnosis	Management
X-linked (Bruton) agammaglobulinemia	- X-linked defect in bruton tyrosine kinase (BTK) - Impaired B-cell maturation	- Recurrent infections by age 3 - 6 months - Scant/absent lymphoid tissue	- Decreased levels of all immunoglobulins - Absent CD19+ B-cells - Normal/high T-cells	- Lifelong immunoglobulin replacement therapy - Prophylactic antibiotics
Common variable immunodeficiency	- Impaired B-cell differentiation	- Recurrent infections during puberty or early adulthood - Associated with chronic pulmonary, gastrointestinal, and autoimmune diseases - Increased risk for malignancy (e.g. lymphoma)	- Markedly decreased levels of IgG - Decreased levels of other immunoglobulins - Normal B-cell and T-cell count - Decreased plasma cell count	- Lifelong immunoglobulin replacement therapy
Selective IgA deficiency	- Isolated deficiency of IgA	- Asymptomatic - Recurrent infections at mucosal surfaces (e.g. lungs, GI) - Chronic giardiasis common	- Decreased levels of IgA - Normal levels of other immunoglobulins - Normal B-cell and T-cell count	- Treat infections - "Wash" pRBCs prior to transfusions

TABLE 18.1.10 - Congenital B Cell Immunodeficiencies

REVIEW QUESTIONS

1. What are the similarities and differences in clinical presentation between X-linked agammaglobulinemia and transient hypogammaglobulinemia of infancy?
    - **Both conditions may present with recurrent sinopulmonary infections and low levels of IgG around 6 months of age.**
    - Patients with transient hypogammaglobulinemia of infancy will have a normal B-cell count, a normal response to immunizations, and they often have some form of atopic disease, such as eczema.
    - Patients with X-linked agammaglobulinemia, on the other hand, will have a decreased B-cell count, no response to immunizations, and have no association with atopic diseases.
    - X-linked agammaglobulinemia is a lifelong condition requiring lifelong immunoglobulin replacement therapy, while the immunoglobulin deficiency in transient hypogammaglobulinemia of infancy will self-resolve and will not require any intervention beyond standard observation.

2. What are the key similarities and differences in clinical presentation of X-linked agammaglobulinemia and common variable immunodeficiency?
    - **Both conditions are characterized by recurrent infections and decreased levels of all immunoglobulins.**
    - X-linked agammaglobulinemia normally presents by age 3 - 6 months, whereas common variable immunodeficiency usually presents during puberty or early adulthood.
    - Additionally, patients with X-linked agammaglobulinemia will have a decreased B-cell count, whereas patients with common variable immunodeficiency will have a normal B-cell count.

3. In a patient with a selective IgA deficiency, what are the main clinical features of an anaphylactic reaction to a blood transfusion?
    - **The main clinical features of an anaphylactic reaction to a blood transfusion are angioedema or urticaria, respiratory distress, and shock within seconds to minutes of receiving a blood transfusion.**

4. A 14-year-old boy is brought to the emergency department by his father due to cough and high fever for the past 24 hours. The boy says he's been coughing up yellow phlegm and has been feeling unwell since yesterday. Past medical history is notable for asthma, recurrent ear infections, and several episodes of giardiasis. Blood pressure is 125/82 mmHg, pulse is 91 beats/minute, respiratory rate is 18 breaths/minute, and temperature is 101.1° F (). Physical examination shows increased work of breathing and crackles on auscultation of the right lower lobe. A chest X-ray confirms the diagnosis of pneumonia, and the patient is admitted for antibiotic therapy. Which of the following is the likely explanation for this patient's recurrent infections?

    A. Decreased T-cell count
    B. Impaired differentiation of B-cells
    C. Decreased B-cell count
    D. Impaired maturation of B-cells

    - **The correct answer is option B.**
    - This is a case of a 14-year-old boy who was admitted to the hospital with a diagnosis of pneumonia.
    - His past medical history is notable for asthma, recurrent ear infections, and several episodes of giardiasis.
    - Given these clinical clues, the most likely explanation for his recurrent infections is an underlying diagnosis of common variable immunodeficiency, which is characterized by failure of mature B-cells to differentiation into plasma cells, impairing production of all immunoglobulins, and creating a state of immunodeficiency.
    - Common variable immunodeficiency typically presents during puberty or early adulthood, and patients also often suffer from chronic lung disease, such as asthma or bronchiectasis.
    - Option A, decreased T-cell count, is incorrect because patients with common variable immunodeficiency have a normal T-cell count.
    - Option C, decreased B-cell count, and option D, impaired maturation of B-cells, are both incorrect because they are features of X-linked agammaglobulinemia, not common variable immunodeficiency.

Pediatrics | Section 15: Congenital T Cell Immunodeficiencies - DiGeorge Syndrome

I. DiGeorge Syndrome: Definition
   A. Congenital disorder that stems from a microdeletion of chromosome 22

II. DiGeorge Syndrome: Pathophysiology
   A. *22q11.2* microdeletion leads to abnormal development of the pharyngeal pouches
      1. Abnormal development of the 3rd pharyngeal pouch leads to thymic aplasia
      2. Thymic aplasia leads to T-cell deficiency

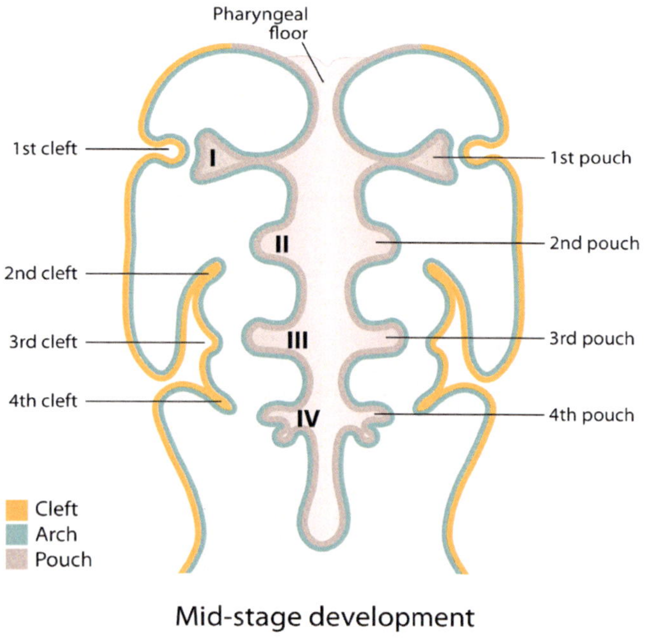

FIGURE 18.1.53 - Pharyngeal Pouches, Clefts, and Arches

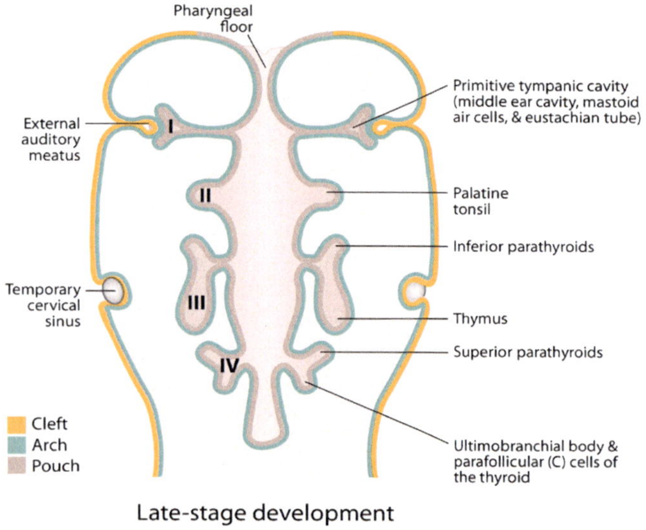

FIGURE 18.1.54 - The Pharyngeal Apparatus

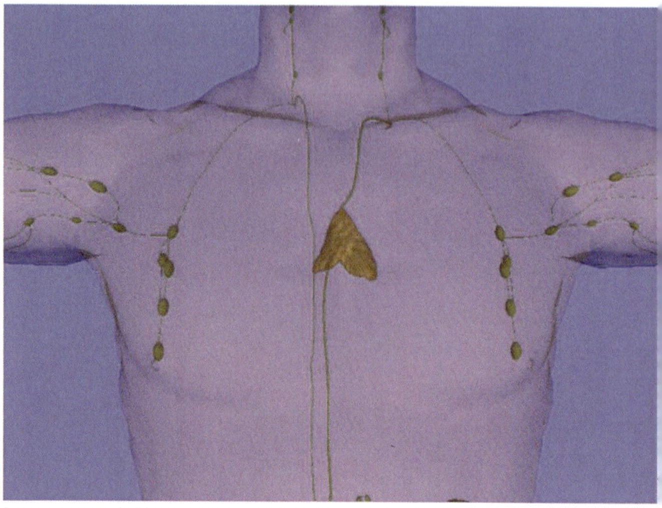

FIGURE 18.1.55 - The Thymus

III. DiGeorge Syndrome: Risk Factors
   A. None
      1. DiGeorge syndrome arises from de novo mutations

IV. DiGeorge Syndrome: Clinical Features
   A. CATCH-22
      1. <u>C</u>left palate
      2. <u>A</u>bnormal facial features (e.g. low-set ears, hypertelorism)
      3. <u>T</u>hymic aplasia
      4. <u>C</u>ardiac defects
      5. <u>H</u>ypoparathyroidism

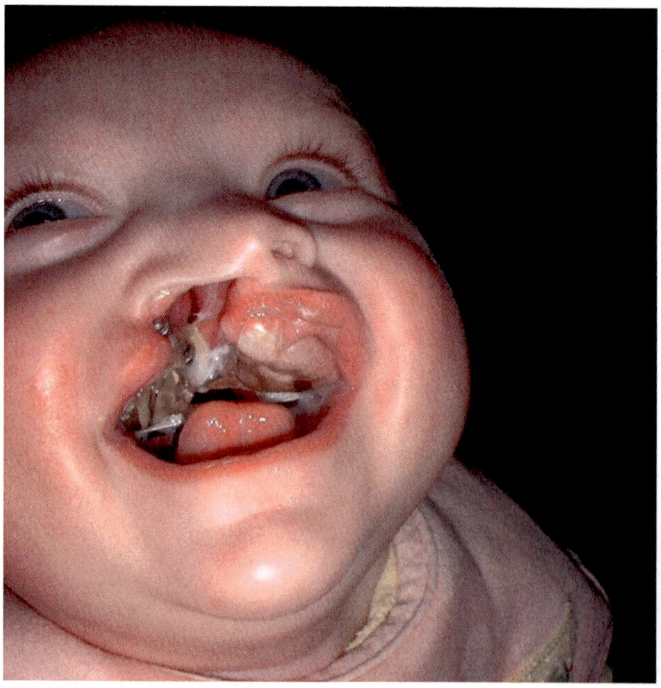

FIGURE 18.1.56 - Cleft Palate

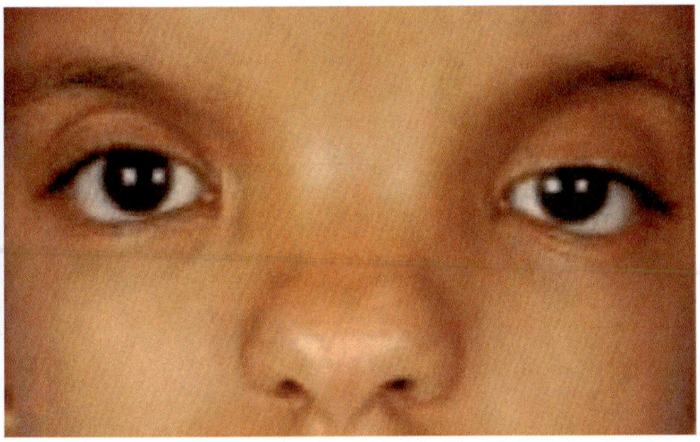

FIGURE 18.1.57 - Hypertelorism

V. DiGeorge Syndrome: Thymic Aplasia
   A. T-cell deficiency
      1. Recurrent infections
      2. Failure to thrive
   B. Absent thymic shadow on X-ray

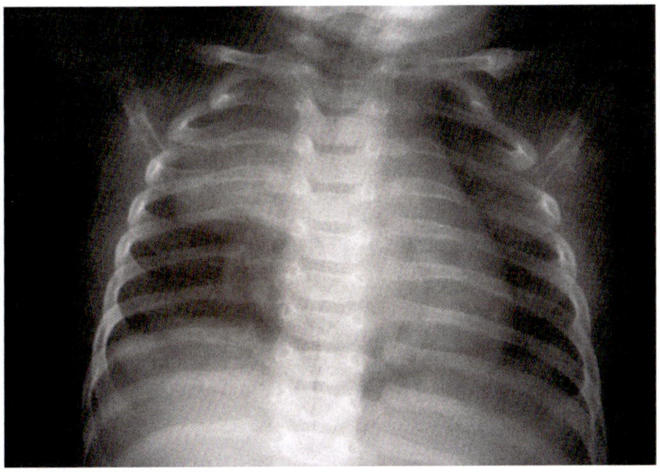

FIGURE 18.1.58 - Chest X-ray of a Healthy Infant

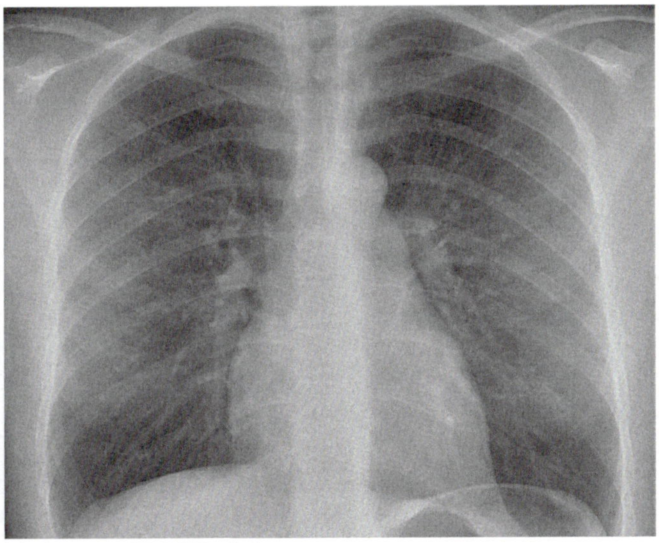

FIGURE 18.1.59 - Chest X-ray of a Healthy Adult

VI. DiGeorge Syndrome: Cardiac Defects
   A. Common defects: truncus arteriosus, tetralogy of fallot
   B. Clinical presentation: cyanosis refractory to supplemental oxygen

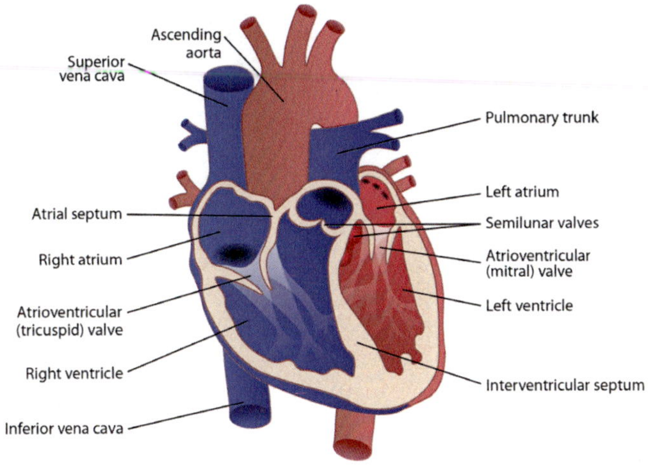

FIGURE 18.1.60 - Normal Heart

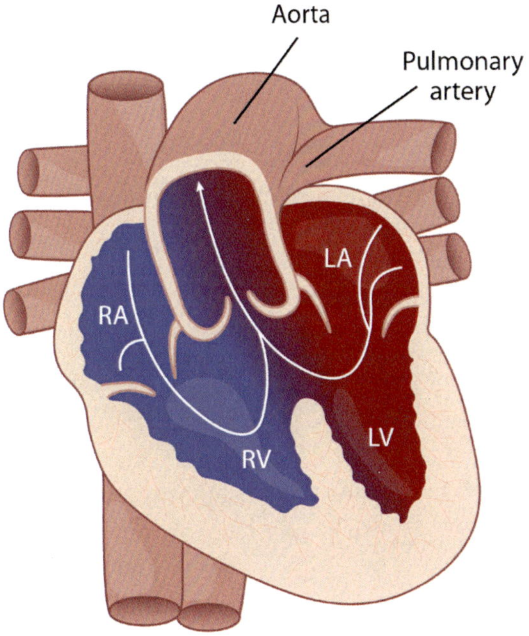

FIGURE 18.1.61 - Truncus Arteriosus

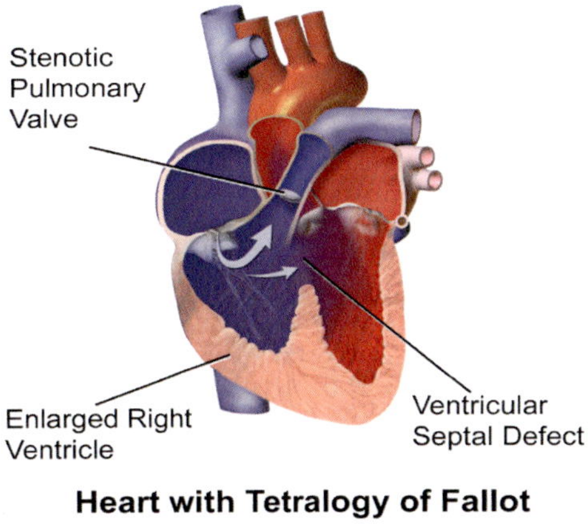

FIGURE 18.1.62 - Tetralogy of Fallot

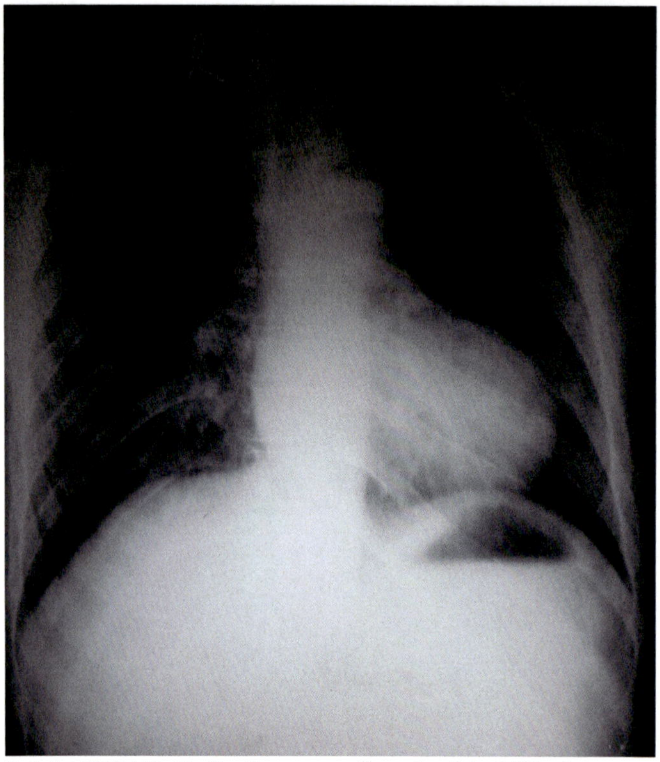

FIGURE 18.1.63 - Chest X-ray: "Boot-Shaped" Heart in Tetralogy of Fallot

VII. DiGeorge Syndrome: Hypoparathyroidism
   A. Hypocalcemia
      1. Seizures
      2. Tetany
      3. Arrhythmias

VIII. DiGeorge Syndrome: Diagnosis
   A. Laboratory evaluation
      1. Low serum PTH and Ca
      2. Lymphopenia
   B. Echocardiography
   C. Fluorescent in situ hybridization (FISH)
      1. Detects *22q11* microdeletion

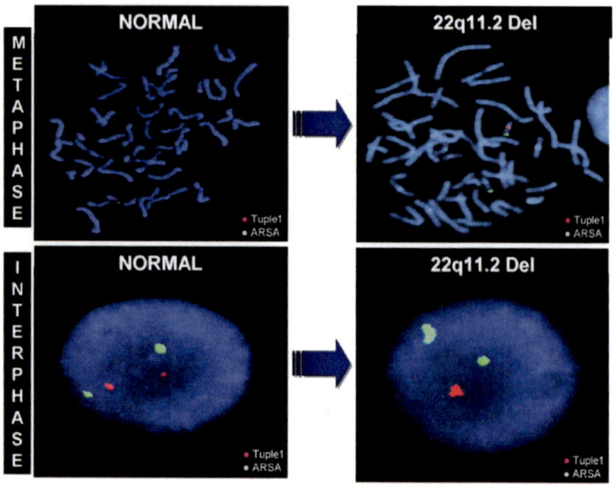

FIGURE 18.1.64 - Fluorescence In-Situ Hybridization: Normal Cells vs Cells with *22q11.2* Microdeletion

IX. DiGeorge Syndrome: Management
   A. Supportive therapy (e.g. treat hypocalcemia)
   B. Age-appropriate vaccinations to prevent infection
   C. Cultured thymic transplant may be curative of immunodeficiency
   D. Surgical correction of craniofacial defects (e.g. cleft palate)
   E. Cardiac surgery to correct cardiac defects

Immunodeficiency	Pathophysiology	Key Features	Diagnosis	Management
DiGeorge syndrome	- *22q11.2* microdeletion - Abnormal development of pharyngeal pouches	- **C**left palate - **A**bnormal facial features - **T**hymic aplasia - **C**ardiac defects - **H**ypoparathyroidism	- Low serum PTH and Ca - Lymphopenia - FISH detects microdeletion	- Age-appropriate vaccinations - Cultured thymic transplant - Surgery for craniofacial and cardiac defects

TABLE 18.1.11 - DiGeorge Syndrome

REVIEW QUESTIONS

1. What are the five key clinical features seen in patients with DiGeorge syndrome?
    - **The five key clinical features seen in patients with DiGeorge syndrome are cleft palate, abnormal facial features, thymic aplasia, cardiac defects, and hypoparathyroidism or hypocalcemia (CATCH-22).**
    - The number 22 in the mnemonic CATCH-22 means that all of this happens due to a microdeletion on chromosome 22.

2. A newborn boy is being evaluated shortly after being born to a 25-year-old mother at 39 weeks gestation via a cesarean delivery for nonreassuring fetal heart tones. The boy is cyanotic, and pulse oximetry shows 82% despite supplemental oxygen therapy. Physical examination shows a cleft palate, widely-spaced eyes, and a holosystolic blowing murmur on auscultation of the heart. A chest X-ray is obtained and shows a "boot-shaped" heart and an absent thymic shadow. An echocardiogram is ordered. Which of the following laboratory findings would be consistent with the patient's most likely underlying diagnosis?

    A. Lymphocytosis
    B. Hypercalcemia
    C. Low serum PTH
    D. Low serum TSH
    E. High serum IgE
    F. High serum PTH

- **The correct answer is option C.**
- This is a case of a newborn boy who is being evaluated for nonreassuring fetal heart tones after being born at 39 weeks gestation via a cesarean delivery.
- The boy is cyanotic and has poor oxygen saturation on pulse oximetry despite supplemental oxygen therapy.
- Physical examination shows a cleft palate, widely-spaced eyes, and a holosystolic blowing murmur.
- These features, in combination with his cyanosis that is refractory to supplemental oxygen, are strongly suggestive of a congenital heart defect.
- Chest X-ray shows a "boot-shaped" heart and an absent thymic shadow, which is suggestive of DiGeorge syndrome in combination with his other symptoms.
- Patients with DiGeorge syndrome often have low serum PTH and calcium as a result of congenital hypoparathyroidism.
- Option A, lymphocytosis, is incorrect because patients with DiGeorge syndrome will likely experience lymphopenia due to a maldeveloped thymus.
- Option B, hypercalcemia, is incorrect because hypoparathyroidism seen in patients with DiGeorge syndrome will lead to hypocalcemia, not hypercalcemia.
- Option D, low serum TSH, is incorrect because thyroid issues are not commonly a part of DiGeorge syndrome.
- Option E, high serum IgE, is incorrect because this is usually a characteristic of Job syndrome, not DiGeorge syndrome.
- Option F, high serum PTH, is incorrect because patients with DiGeorge syndrome experience hypoparathyroidism, not hyperparathyroidism.

Pediatrics | Section 16: Continental T-Cell Immunodeficiencies - Job Syndrome, IPEX Syndrome & Chronic Mucocutaneous Disease

I. Job Syndrome: Definition
  A. Primary immunodeficiency characterized by elevated levels of IgE
  B. Also known as Hyper-IgE syndrome

II. Job Syndrome: Pathophysiology
  A. Autosomal dominant genetic mutation
    1. Causes overproduction of IgE
    2. Impairs T-cell function and neutrophil chemotaxis

III. Job Syndrome: Risk Factors
  A. Family history

IV. Job Syndrome: Clinical Features
  A. Classic triad
    1. Atopic dermatitis
    2. Recurrent pulmonary infections
    3. Recurrent skin infections (particularly with *S. aureus*)
  B. Facial abnormalities (e.g. deep-set eyes, broad nasal bridge)
  C. Musculoskeletal abnormalities (e.g. osteopenia, scoliosis)

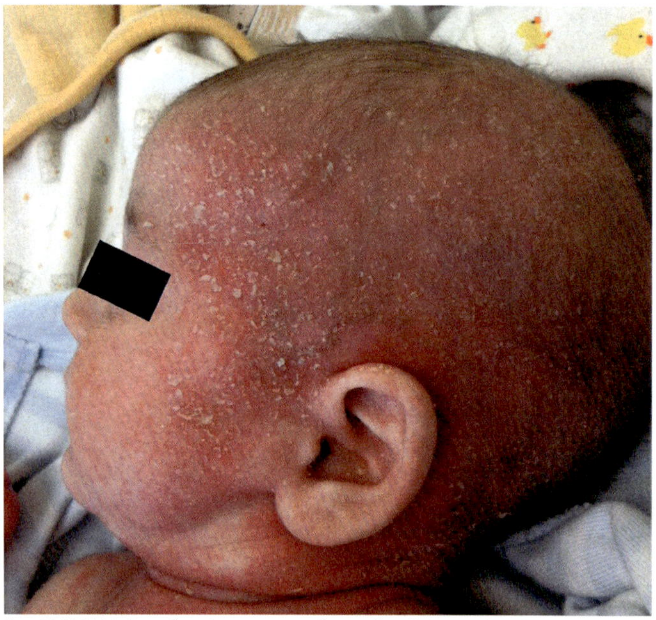

FIGURE 18.1.65 - Atopic Dermatitis

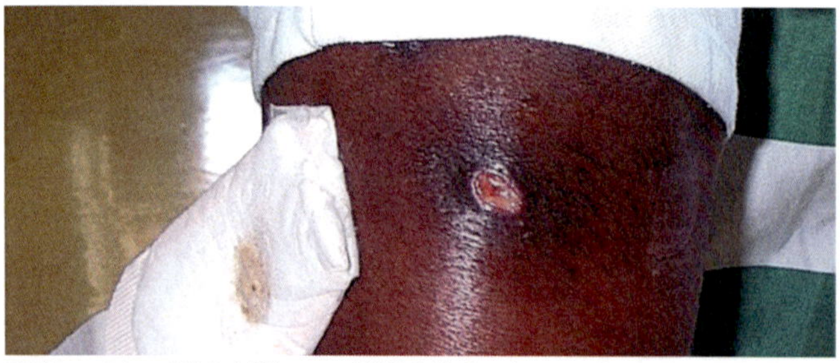

FIGURE 18.1.66 - A Cutaneous Abscess

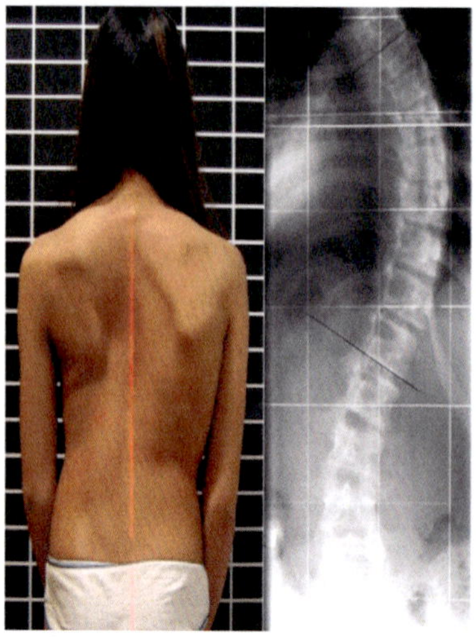

FIGURE 18.1.67 - Scoliosis

V. Job Syndrome: Diagnosis
  A. Laboratory evaluation
    1. Very high levels of IgE
    2. Normal levels of other immunoglobulins (e.g. IgA, IgG, IgM)
    3. Eosinophilia
  B. Genetic testing may confirm diagnosis

VI. Job Syndrome: Management
  A. No cure
  B. Treat recurrent infections
    1. Consider prophylactic antibiotics
  C. Treat musculoskeletal abnormalities (e.g. scoliosis)

VII. IPEX Syndrome: Definition
  A. Immunodeficiency syndrome characterized by:
    1. **I**mmune dysregulation
    2. **P**olyendocrinopathy
    3. **E**nteropathy
    4. **X**-linked inheritance

VIII. IPEX Syndrome: Pathophysiology
  A. Genetic mutation impairs function of regulatory T-cells
    1. Regulatory T-cells suppress the immune system
    2. Impairment of regulatory T-cells results in autoimmune reactions

IX. IPEX Syndrome: Risk Factors
  A. Male sex

X. IPEX Syndrome: Clinical Features
  A. Clinical triad
    1. Eczematous dermatitis
    2. Enteropathy (e.g. watery diarrhea)
    3. Endocrinopathy (e.g. type 1 diabetes mellitus)
  B. Autoimmune phenomena (e.g. cytopenias, arthritis)

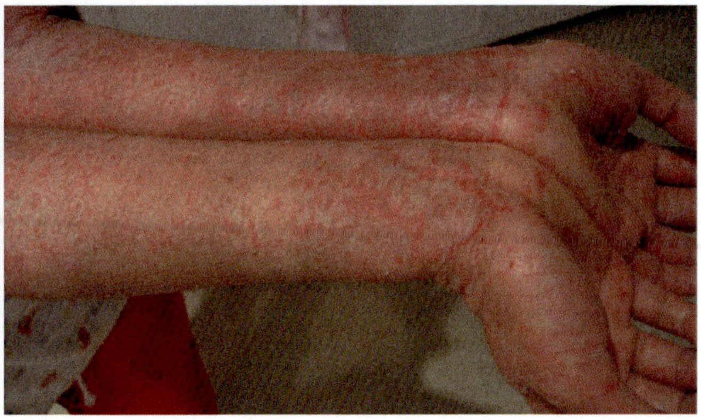

FIGURE 18.1.68 - Eczematous Dermatitis

XI. IPEX Syndrome: Diagnosis
   A. Genetic testing

XII. IPEX Syndrome: Management
   A. Immunosuppressive therapy (e.g. steroids)
   B. Supportive treatment (e.g. treat diabetes mellitus)
   C. Bone marrow transplant may be curative

XIII. Chronic Mucocutaneous Candidiasis: Definition
   A. Chronic, recurrent superficial *Candida* infections of skin, nails, and mucous membranes

XIV. Chronic Mucocutaneous Candidiasis: Pathophysiology
   A. Autosomal recessive mutation disrupts
      1. T-cell function
      2. Regulation of autoimmune reactions

XV. Chronic Mucocutaneous Candidiasis: Risk Factors
   A. Family history

XVI. Chronic Mucocutaneous Candidiasis: Clinical Features
   A. Recurrent, superficial infections with *Candida* species
   B. Autoimmune manifestations (e.g. cytopenias, endocrinopathies)
      1. Common endocrinopathies: type 1 diabetes mellitus and hypoparathyroidism

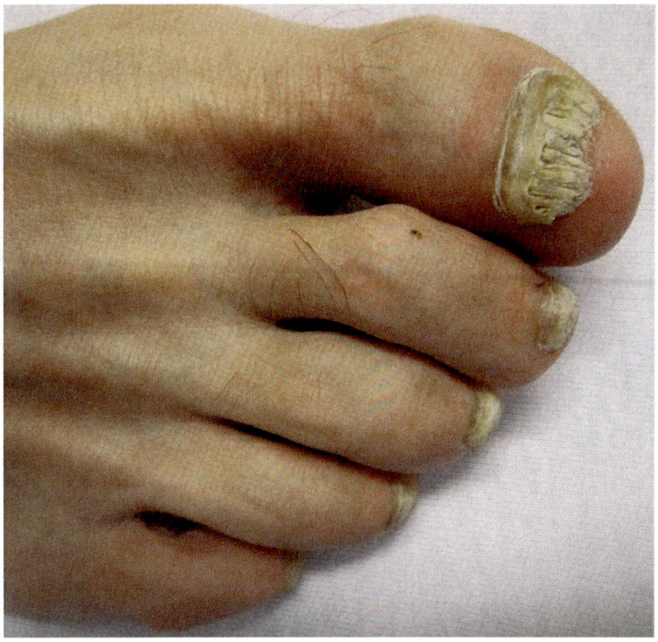

FIGURE 18.1.69 - Onychomycosis

XVII. Chronic Mucocutaneous Candidiasis: Diagnosis
   A. Clinical diagnosis
   B. Genetic testing

XVIII. Chronic Mucocutaneous Candidiasis: Management
   A. Treat recurrent infections
      1. Antifungal medications (e.g. azoles)
   B. Treat autoimmune manifestations and endocrinopathies

Immunodeficiency	Pathophysiology	Key Features	Diagnosis	Management
DiGeorge syndrome	- 22q11.2 microdeletion - Abnormal development of pharyngeal pouches	- **C**left palate - **A**bnormal facial features - **T**hymic aplasia - **C**ardiac defects - **H**ypoparathyroidism	- Low serum PTH and Ca - Lymphopenia - FISH detects microdeletion	- Age-appropriate vaccinations - Cultured thymic transplant - Surgery for craniofacial and cardiac defects
Job (Hyper-IgE) syndrome	- Autosomal dominant mutation - Impaired T-cell function - Impaired neutrophil chemotaxis - Overproduction of IgE	- Atopic dermatitis - Recurrent pulmonary and skin infections - Facial abnormalities - Musculoskeletal abnormalities	- Elevated IgE - Eosinophilia - Genetic testing to confirm diagnosis	- No cure - Treat recurrent infections - Treat musculoskeletal abnormalities
IPEX syndrome	- X-linked recessive mutation - Impaired regulatory T-cells	- Eczematous dermatitis - Enteropathy (e.g. watery diarrhea) - Endocrinopathy (e.g. T1DM) - Autoimmune phenomena	- Genetic testing to confirm diagnosis	- Immunosuppressive therapy - Bone marrow transplant may be curative
Chronic mucocutaneous candidiasis	- Autosomal recessive mutation - Impaired T-cell function - Impaired regulation of autoimmune reactions	- Recurrent superficial *Candida* infections - Autoimmune manifestations	- Clinical diagnosis - Genetic testing confirms diagnosis	- Treat recurrent infections (e.g. using azoles) - Treat autoimmune manifestations

TABLE 18.1.12 - Congenital T-Cell Immunodeficiencies

REVIEW QUESTIONS

1. What is the classic triad of symptoms that characterizes Job (Hyper-IgE) syndrome?
    - **The classic triad of symptoms that characterizes Job (Hyper-IgE) syndrome are atopic dermatitis, recurrent pulmonary infections, and recurrent skin infections.**
    - These findings will almost always be accompanied by very high levels of serum IgE.
2. What is the classic triad of symptoms that characterizes IPEX syndrome?
    - **The classic triad of symptoms that characterizes IPEX syndrome includes eczematous dermatitis, enteropathy, which often manifests in the form of watery diarrhea, and endocrinopathy, such as type 1 diabetes mellitus.**
3. A 12-year-old girl is brought to the emergency department by her mother because of concern for a "leg infection." The mother says that the girl sustained a minor cut while playing in their backyard yesterday. Since then, the girl developed a low-grade fever and pain in the left shin. She has a history of atopic dermatitis, mild scoliosis, recurrent skin infections, and two prior hospitalizations for pneumonia. Blood pressure is 105/75 mmHg, pulse is 85 beats/minute, and temperature is 101.1° F (38.4° C). Physical examination shows a small cut on the left anterior shin that is oozing yellow-brown fluid and feels fluctuant to palpation. The girl is also noted to have deep-set eyes and a broad nasal bridge. Initial laboratory evaluation shows eosinophilia and elevated levels of IgE. Which of the following is the most likely diagnosis?

    A. DiGeorge syndrome
    B. Job syndrome
    C. IPEX syndrome
    D. Chronic mucocutaneous candidiasis

    - **The correct answer is option B.**
    - This 12-year-old girl presents with low-grade fever and pain in the left shin.
    - She has a history of atopic dermatitis, scoliosis, recurrent skin infections, and prior hospitalizations for pneumonia.
    - During the examination, she has a fever at 38.4° C (101.1° F) and a cut on the left anterior shin that is oozing yellow-brown fluid and feels fluctuant to palpation, which suggests that the girl may have developed an abscess.
    - Her labs are notable for eosinophilia and elevated levels of IgE.
    - All of these key clinical features are consistent with Job syndrome or Hyper-IgE syndrome, which is why option B is the correct answer.
    - Option A is incorrect because DiGeorge syndrome is unlikely as it is not commonly associated with atopic dermatitis, scoliosis, or elevated levels of IgE.
    - Option C is incorrect because IPEX syndrome is not commonly associated with facial abnormalities like deep-set eyes or elevated levels of IgE. Furthermore, IPEX syndrome is an X-linked recessive disorder, which makes it uncommon among girls.
    - Option D, chronic mucocutaneous candidiasis, is unlikely because this girl does not have a prior history of *Candida* infections.

Pediatrics | Section 17: Congenital Mixed Immunodeficiencies: Severe Combined Immunodeficiency & Wiskott Aldrich Syndrome

I. Severe Combined Immunodeficiency: Definition
   A. Primary immunodeficiency disorder of T-cells and B-cells

II. Severe Combined Immunodeficiency: Pathophysiology
   A. Genetic mutation disrupts T-cell maturation and function
      1. X-linked recessive defect in interleukin receptors
      2. Autosomal recessive defect in adenosine deaminase (ADA)
   B. Impairment of T-cells causes dysfunction of B-cells

III. Severe Combined Immunodeficiency: Risk Factors
   A. Male sex
   B. Family history

IV. Severe Combined Immunodeficiency: Clinical Features
   A. Recurrent infections that start by age six months
      1. Viral
      2. Fungal (e.g. *Candida* thrush)
      3. Opportunistic (e.g. *Pneumocystis jirovecii* pneumonia)
   B. Chronic diarrhea
   C. Failure to thrive
   D. Scant lymph tissue on physical exam (e.g. Tonsils, lymph nodes)

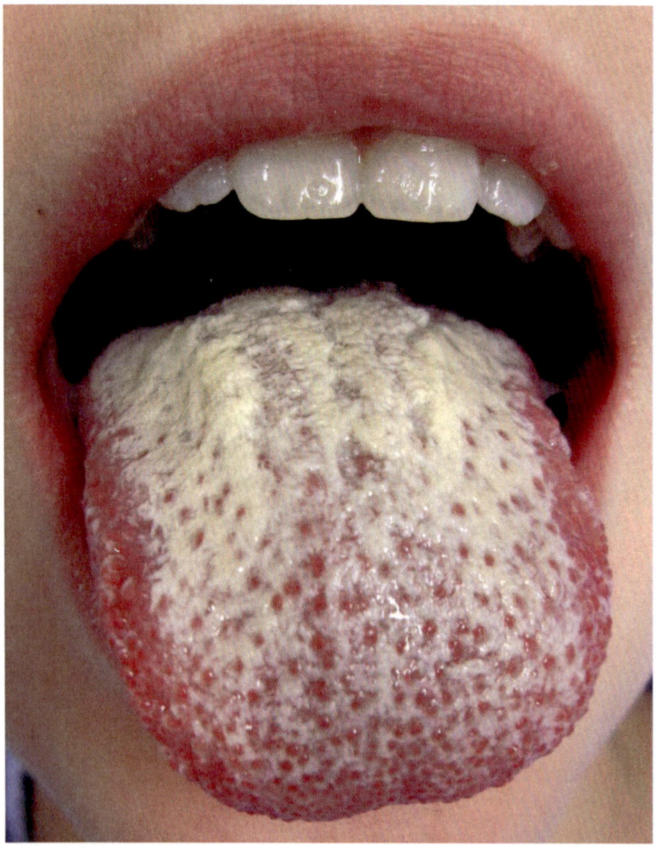

FIGURE 18.1.70 - Patient with Oral Thrush Due to Infection with *Candida*

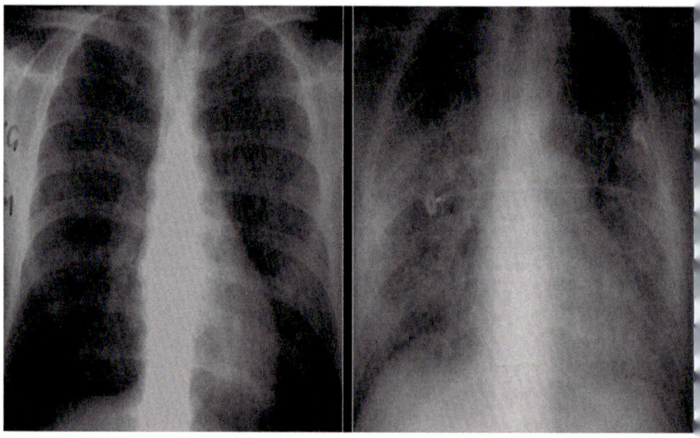

FIGURE 18.1.71 - Chest X-ray Showing Bilateral "Ground-Glass"

V. Severe Combined Immunodeficiency: Diagnosis
   A. Newborn screening
      1. Absence of T-cell receptor excision circles
   B. Flow cytometry
      1. Markedly decreased T-cell and B-cell counts
   C. Quantitative serum immunoglobulin measurement
      1. Decreased levels of all immunoglobulins (e.g. IgA, IgG)
   D. Absence of thymic shadow on chest X-ray

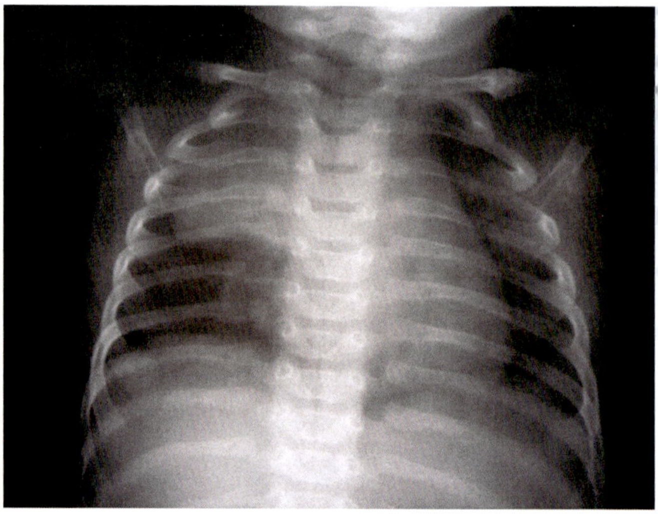

FIGURE 18.1.72 - Healthy Baby Chest X-Ray

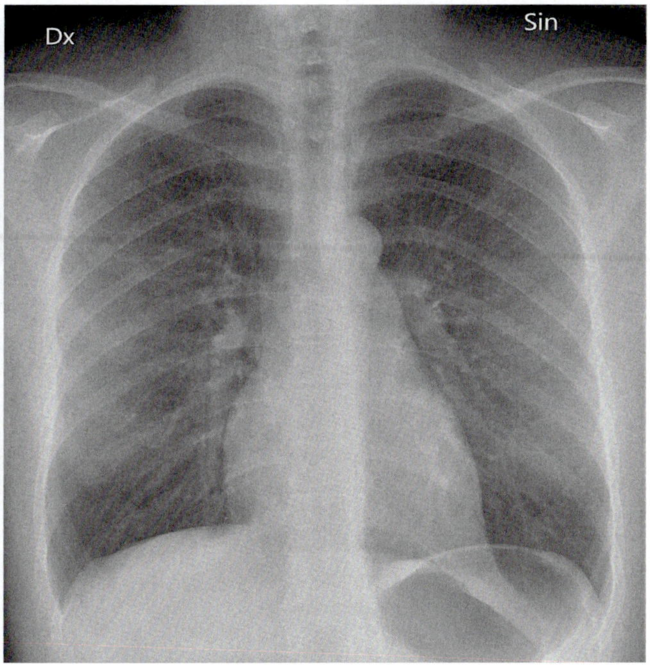

FIGURE 18.1.73 - Healthy Adult Chest X-Ray

1. Severe Combined Immunodeficiency: Management
   E. Stem cell transplant is the only definitive/long-term treatment
      1. Consider antibiotic prophylaxis and/or IVIG transfusions while awaiting a stem cell transplant
   F. Avoid live vaccines
      1. Inactivated vaccines will not be effective

VI. Wiskott-Aldrich Syndrome: Definition
   A. Primary immunodeficiency disorder that affects leukocytes and platelets

VII. Wiskott-Aldrich Syndrome: Pathophysiology
   A. X-linked recessive mutation in WAS gene impairs cytoskeleton remodeling/regulation of leukocytes and platelets

VIII. Wiskott Aldrich Syndrome: Risk Factors
   A. Male sex

IX. Wiskott Aldrich Syndrome: Clinical Features
   A. Presents early in infancy
   B. Classic triad
      1. Recurrent infections
      2. Eczema
      3. Microthrombocytopenia (e.g. bleeding, bruising, petechiae/purpura)

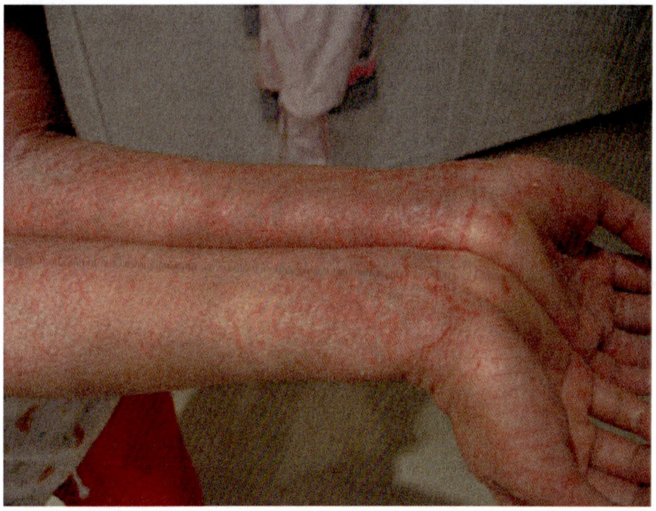

FIGURE 18.1.74 - Eczema in Patient with Wiskott-Aldrich Syndrome

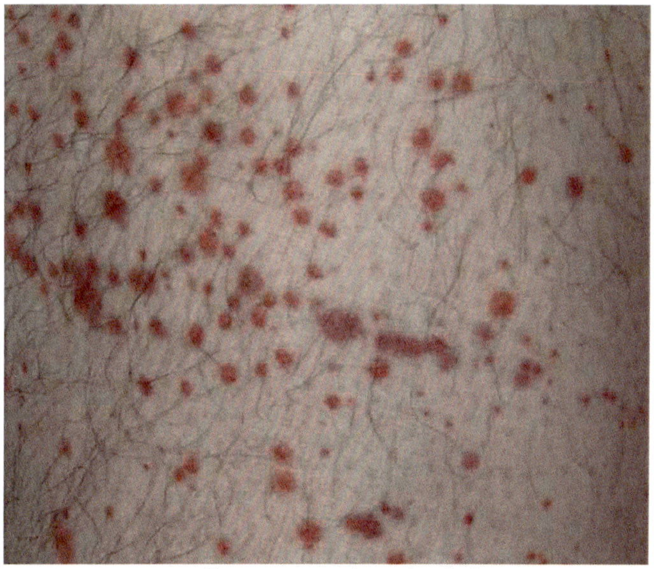

FIGURE 18.1.75 - Petechiae and Purpura in Patients with Thrombocytopenia

X. Wiskott Aldrich Syndrome: Diagnosis
   A. CBC: thrombocytopenia +/- lymphopenia
   B. Quantitative serum immunoglobulin measurement
      1. Elevated IgA and IgE
      2. Decreased IgG and IgM
   C. Genetic testing

XI. Wiskott Aldrich Syndrome: Management
   A. Stem cell transplant

Immunodeficiency	Pathophysiology	Key Features	Diagnosis	Management
Severe combined immunodeficiency (SCID)	- X-linked recessive defect in interleukin receptors - Autosomal recessive defect in adenosine deaminase - Dysfunction of T-cells and B-cells	- Recurrent infections by 6 months of age - Opportunistic infections are common (e.g. *Candida*) - Chronic diarrhea - Failure to thrive - Scant lymph tissue on exam	- Newborn screening - Decreased T-cells and B-cells - Decreased immunoglobulins - No thymic shadow on X-ray	- Stem cell transplant is the only definitive treatment - Consider IVIG or prophylactic antibiotics - Avoid live vaccines
Wiskott-Aldrich syndrome	- X-linked recessive mutation in WAS gene - Impaired remodeling/regulation of cytoskeleton in leukocytes and platelets	- Presents in infancy - Triad of recurrent infections, eczema, and microthrombocytopenia	- Thrombocytopenia - Elevated IgA and IgE - Decreased IgG and IgM - Genetic testing	- Stem cell transplant

TABLE 18.1.13 - Severe Combined Immunodeficiency and Wiskott Aldrich Syndrome

REVIEW QUESTIONS

1. How can clinicians distinguish thrush (left) from leukoplakia (right) on physical examination?

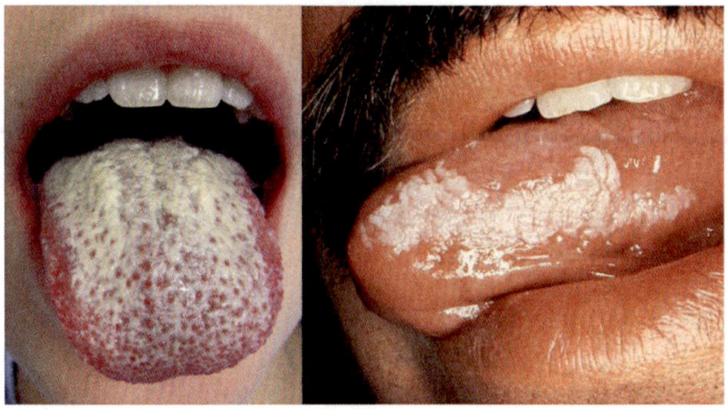

James Heilman, MD, CC BY-SA 3.0 <https://creativecommons.org/licenses/by-sa/3.0>, via Wikimedia Commons

FIGURE 18.1.70 - Thrush

Aitor III, Public domain, via Wikimedia Commons

FIGURE 18.1.76 - Leukoplakia

- **The easiest way to distinguish oral thrush from leukoplakia is to try to scrape the lesion with a tongue depressor. If the patient has thrush, the clinician will be able to scrape the white lesions off the tongue. If the patient has leukoplakia the clinician will not be able to scrape the white lesions off the tongue.**

2. Aside from severe combined immunodeficiency, which additional congenital immunodeficiency disorder may result in an absence of the thymic shadow on chest X-ray of a newborn baby?

- **Absence of thymic shadow on chest X-ray of a newborn baby may be seen in severe combined immunodeficiency and DiGeorge syndrome.**
- DiGeorge syndrome has 5 key clinical features that can be remembered with the CATCH-22 mnemonic.
- The mnemonic stands for cleft palate, abnormal facial features, thymic aplasia, cardiac defects, and hypoparathyroidism or hypocalcemia. The number 22 indicates all of this happens due to a microdeletion on chromosome 22.
- Bearing these clinical features in mind, newborns with DiGeorge syndrome will not have a thymic shadow on chest X-ray due to thymic aplasia.

3. What are the similarities and differences in clinical presentation of severe combined immunodeficiency and HIV in infancy?

- **Severe combined immunodeficiency and HIV in infancy will have several clinical features in common: chronic diarrhea, failure to thrive, and opportunistic infections, most commonly with *Pneumocystis* or *Candida.***
- **For differences, babies with severe combined immunodeficiency will have lymphopenia, whereas babies with HIV in infancy will have a normal absolute lymphocyte count but a low $CD4^+$ T-cell count.**
- **Patients with SCID will have no lymphadenopathy or hepatosplenomegaly, whereas babies with HIV in infancy will likely have lymphadenopathy and potentially hepatosplenomegaly.**

4. What is the triad of clinical features often seen in patients with Wiskott-Aldrich syndrome?

- **The classic triad of clinical features seen in patients with Wiskott-Aldrich syndrome is recurrent infections, eczema, and microthrombocytopenia.**

REVIEW QUESTIONS

5. A 4-month-old girl is brought to the primary care physician by her mom because of a "white rash on her tongue." She has a history of chronic diarrhea, multiple episodes of otitis media, and a prior hospitalization for pneumonia. Temperature is 98.8° F (37.1° C) and pulse is 100 beats/minute. The girl is at the second percentile for weight. Physical examination shows white, fluffy lesions on the girl's tongue that can be scraped off with a tongue depressor. There are no visible tonsils and the lymph nodes are not palpable. Laboratory evaluation shows a decreased absolute lymphocyte count and decreased serum levels of all immunoglobulins. Which of the following additional findings would be consistent with this patient's most likely underlying diagnosis?

    A. Elevated alpha-fetoprotein
    B. Thrombocytopenia
    C. Absent thymic shadow on chest X-ray
    D. A history of eczema
    E. Absent CD40 ligand on flow cytometry
    F. A positive HIV test

- **The correct answer is option C.**
- This is a case of a 4-month-old girl who is brought to the pediatrician with a white rash on her tongue which can be scraped off with a tongue depressor.
- This should instantly raise suspicion for oral thrush which, in turn, should raise suspicion for a congenital immunodeficiency, especially given the history of chronic diarrhea, multiple episodes of otitis media, a prior hospitalization for pneumonia, and failure to thrive.
- Furthermore, this girl's physical examination shows no visible tonsils and no palpable lymph nodes, and her laboratory evaluation reveals a decrease in the absolute lymphocyte count and all immunoglobulins.
- Putting all of these clues together, this girl's most likely underlying diagnosis is severe combined immunodeficiency.
- The clinical features of severe combined immunodeficiency include recurrent viral, fungal, and opportunistic infections that start by age six months, chronic diarrhea, failure to thrive, and scant lymph tissue on physical examination, such as absent tonsils or non-palpable lymph nodes. The patient in question had all of these clinical features.
- One of the key diagnostic features of severe combined immunodeficiency is the absence of thymic shadow on chest X-ray.
- Option A is incorrect because elevated alpha-fetoprotein is not seen in patients with SCID. Rather, it can be seen in patients with ataxia-telangiectasia syndrome.
- Option B, thrombocytopenia, and option D, a history of eczema, are both clinical features of Wiskott-Aldrich syndrome, which is unlikely in this clinical vignette.
- First, Wiskott-Aldrich syndrome is X-linked recessive and is, therefore, more commonly seen in boys than in girls.
- Second, this patient does not have any clinical features that would indicate a thrombocytopenia, such as petechiae, purpura, and history of bleeding or easy bruising.
- And third, absence of tonsils and palpable lymph nodes is not a common clinical feature of Wiskott-Aldrich syndrome.
- Option E is incorrect because absent CD40 ligand on flow cytometry is a feature of hyper-IgM syndrome, not SCID. Hyper-IgM syndrome is unlikely in this patient because her laboratory evaluation revealed decreased serum levels of all immunoglobulins. Patients with Hyper-IgM syndrome would have elevated levels of IgM.
- Option F is incorrect because infants with HIV usually have lymphadenopathy and potentially hepatosplenomegaly, rather than absent or scant lymph tissue.

Pediatrics | Section 18: Congenital Mixed Immunodeficiencies - Hyper-IgM Syndrome & Ataxia-Telangiectasia

I. Hyper-IgM Syndrome: Definition
   A. Primary immunodeficiency disorder characterized by elevated levels of IgM and diminished levels of other immunoglobulins

II. Hyper-IgM Syndrome: Pathophysiology
   A. X-linked recessive mutation causes a deficiency of CD40 ligand on T-cells
   B. CD40 ligand is necessary for:
      1. Class-switching of B-cells
      2. Formation of memory B-cells and long-term immune response

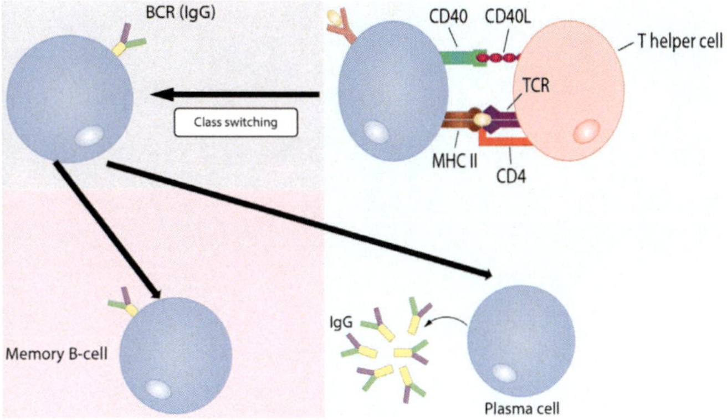

FIGURE 18.1.77 - Class Switching of B Cells

III. Hyper-IgM Syndrome: Risk Factors
   A. Male sex

IV. Hyper-IgM Syndrome: Clinical Features
   A. Presents early in infancy
   B. Recurrent sinopulmonary infections (e.g. otitis media, pneumonia)
      1. Susceptibility to encapsulated organisms (e.g. *S. pneumoniae*)
      2. Susceptibility to opportunistic infections (e.g. *P. jirovecii*)
   C. Failure to thrive
   D. Scant lymph tissue on physical exam (e.g. tonsils, lymph nodes)

V. Hyper-IgM Syndrome: Diagnosis
   A. Quantitative serum immunoglobulin measurement
      1. Elevated IgM
      2. Decreased IgG, IgA, and IgE
   B. Flow cytometry
      1. Absence of CD40 ligand on lymphocytes
   C. Genetic testing

VI. Hyper-IgM Syndrome: Management
   A. Intravenous immunoglobulin therapy
   B. Antibiotic prophylaxis

VII. Ataxia-Telangiectasia: Definition
   A. Primary immunodeficiency syndrome that impairs both T-cells and B-cells
   B. Also known as Louis-Bar syndrome

VIII. Ataxia-Telangiectasia: Pathophysiology
   A. Autosomal recessive mutation in the ATM gene disrupts DNA repair
      1. DNA damage accumulates in lymphocytes, leading to their death

IX. Ataxia-Telangiectasia: Risk Factors
   A. Family history

X. Ataxia-Telangiectasia: Clinical Features
   A. Ataxia (due to progressive cerebellar atrophy)
   B. Telangiectasias on skin and eyes
   C. Abnormal eye movements
   D. Recurrent sinopulmonary infections (e.g. otitis media, pneumonia)
   E. Increased risk for cancer (e.g. lymphoma, leukemia)
   F. Scant lymph tissue on physical exam (e.g. tonsils, lymph nodes)

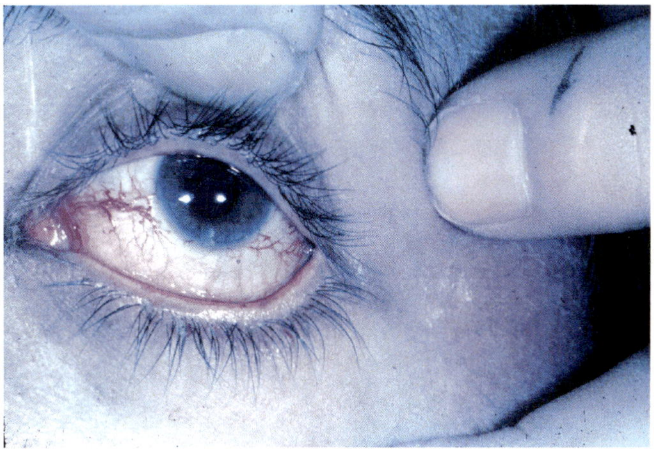

FIGURE 18.1.78 - Ocular Telangiectasias

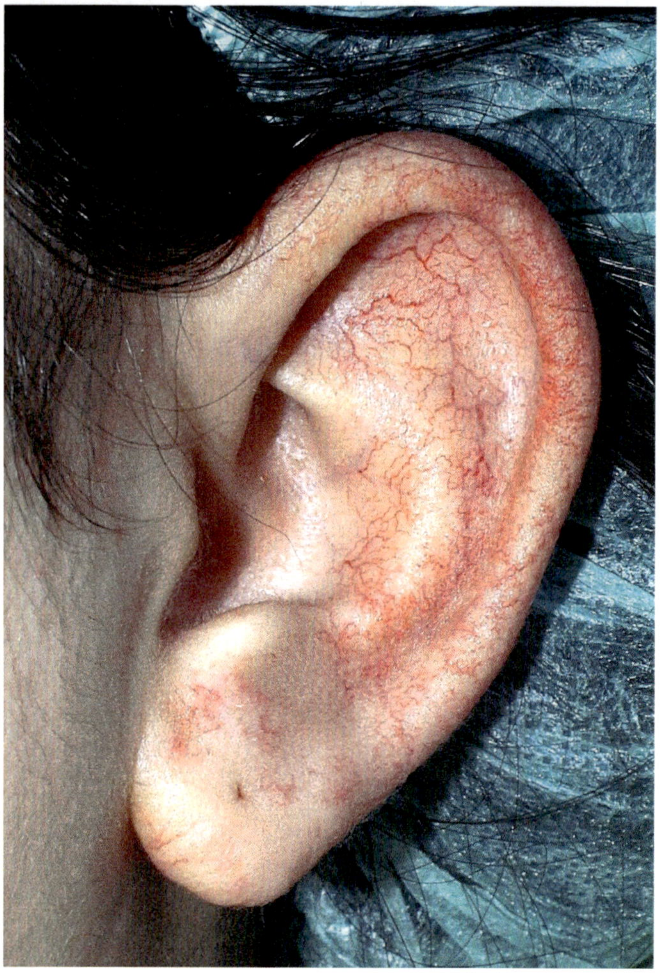

FIGURE 18.1.79 - Cutaneous Telangiectasias

XI. Ataxia-Telangiectasia: Diagnosis
   A. Laboratory evaluation
      1. Elevated AFP
      2. Decreased IgG and IgA
         a. Genetic testing

XII. Ataxia-Telangiectasia: Management
   A. Supportive treatment (e.g. physical therapy)
   B. Intravenous immunoglobulin therapy
   C. Antibiotic prophylaxis
   D. Cancer surveillance

Immunodeficiency	Pathophysiology	Key Features	Diagnosis	Management
Hyper-IgM syndrome	- X-linked recessive mutation causes a deficiency of CD40L - Impaired class-switching - Impaired formation of memory B cells	- Presents in infancy - Recurrent infections - Susceptibility to encapsulated organisms and opportunistic infections - Failure to thrive - Scant lymph tissue on exam	- Elevated IgM - Decreased IgG, IgA, IgE - Absent CD40 ligand on lymphocytes - Genetic testing	- IVIG - Antibiotic prophylaxis
Ataxia-telangiectasia	- Autosomal recessive mutation in ATM gene - Compromised DNA repair	- Ataxia - Telangiectasias - Abnormal eye movements - Recurrent infections - Increased risk for cancer - Scant lymph tissue on exam	- Elevated AFP - Decreased IgG and IgA - Genetic testing	- Supportive treatment (e.g. physical therapy) - IVIG - Antibiotic prophylaxis - Cancer surveillance

TABLE 18.1.14 - Hyper-IgM Syndrome and Ataxia-Telangiectasia

REVIEW QUESTIONS

1. Do patients with Hyper-IgM syndrome benefit from immunizations?
    - **No, patients with Hyper-IgM syndrome will not benefit from immunizations.**
    - This is because these patients have impaired production of immunoglobulins and memory B-cells, preventing them from mounting an adequate immune response to immunizations and subsequent exposure to the vaccine's antigens.

2. A 2-year-old girl is brought to the emergency department by her mother because of a high fever and labored breathing for the past few hours. She has a past medical history of recurrent sinus and ear infections. She had a recent hospitalization for pneumonia. Blood pressure is 105/72 mmHg, pulse is 95 beats/minute, and temperature is 102.2° F (39.0° C). Physical examination shows diffuse crackles throughout both lungs. Lymph nodes are not palpable. Several small, dilated, tortuous blood vessels are notable on the patient's sclera and skin. Initial laboratory evaluation shows lymphopenia. A chest X-ray shows bilateral ground-glass opacities and a tracheal aspirate is positive for *Pneumocystis jirovecii*. Which of the following underlying mechanisms is the most likely cause of this patient's recurrent infections?

    A. Impaired class-switching
    B. Deficiency of CD40 ligand
    C. Mutation in the WAS gene
    D. Mutation in the ATM gene

    - **The correct answer is option D.**
    - This is a case of a 2-year-old girl who has a history of recurrent sinus and ear infections and a recent hospitalization for pneumonia.
    - The lymph nodes are not palpable on physical examination, and lymphopenia is noted on laboratory studies.
    - Tracheal aspirate is positive for *Pneumocystis jirovecii*, an opportunistic pathogen.
    - All of these clues suggest an underlying primary immunodeficiency.
    - There are several small dilated, tortuous blood vessels on the patient's sclera and skin. This is a classic description of telangiectasias.
    - Presence of telangiectasias in the context of a likely primary immunodeficiency syndrome is strongly suggestive of ataxia-telangiectasia as the underlying cause of this girl's recurrent infections
    - Ataxia-telangiectasia is caused by an autosomal recessive mutation in the ATM gene.
    - Option A and option B are incorrect because impaired class-switching and deficiency of CD40 ligand are both features of Hyper-IgM syndrome. Hyper-IgM syndrome is less likely to present with telangiectasias.
    - Option C is incorrect because mutation in the WAS gene is a feature of Wiskott-Aldrich syndrome, which is characterized by a triad of recurrent infections, microthrombocytopenia, and eczema. Telangiectasias are uncommon in Wiskott-Aldrich syndrome.

Pediatrics | Section 19: Congenital Phagocyte Defects - Chronic Granulomatous Disease & Myeloperoxidase Deficiency

I. Chronic Granulomatous Disease: Definition
   A. Primary immunodeficiency syndrome characterized by a defective oxidative burst within phagocytes (e.g. neutrophils, macrophages)

II. Chronic Granulomatous Disease: Pathophysiology
   A. Genetic defect in NADPH oxidase impairs the oxidative burst
      1. Phagocytes become less capable of killing pathogens
   B. X-linked recessive inheritance pattern is most common
      1. Autosomal recessive inheritance pattern is possible

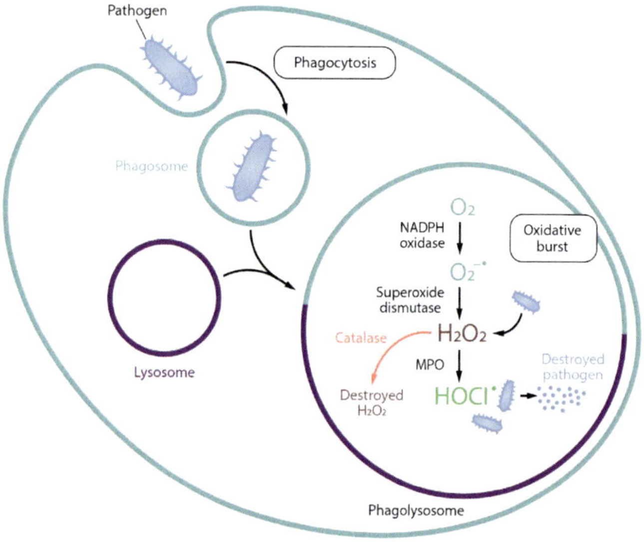

FIGURE 18.1.80 - Pathophysiology of Chronic Granulomatous Disease

III. Chronic Granulomatous Disease: Risk Factors
   A. Male sex
   B. Family history

IV. Chronic Granulomatous Disease: Clinical Features
   A. Recurrent infections with catalase-positive pathogens
      1. Common infections: pneumonia, cutaneous abscess, suppurative adenitis, osteomyelitis
      2. Common pathogens: *S. aureus*, *P. cepacia*, *S. marcescens*, *Aspergillus* species, *Nocardia* species
   B. Granulomas anywhere in the body (e.g. skin, visceral organs)

V. Chronic Granulomatous Disease: Diagnosis
   A. Dihydrorhodamine flow cytometry (gold-standard)
      1. Normal: green fluorescence
      2. Defective NADPH oxidase: diminished green fluorescence
   B. Nitroblue tetrazolium dye test
      1. Normal: dye turns blue
      2. Defective NADPH oxidase: dye remains colorless
   C. Gram stain of phagocytes
      1. Organisms within phagocytes
   D. Genetic testing

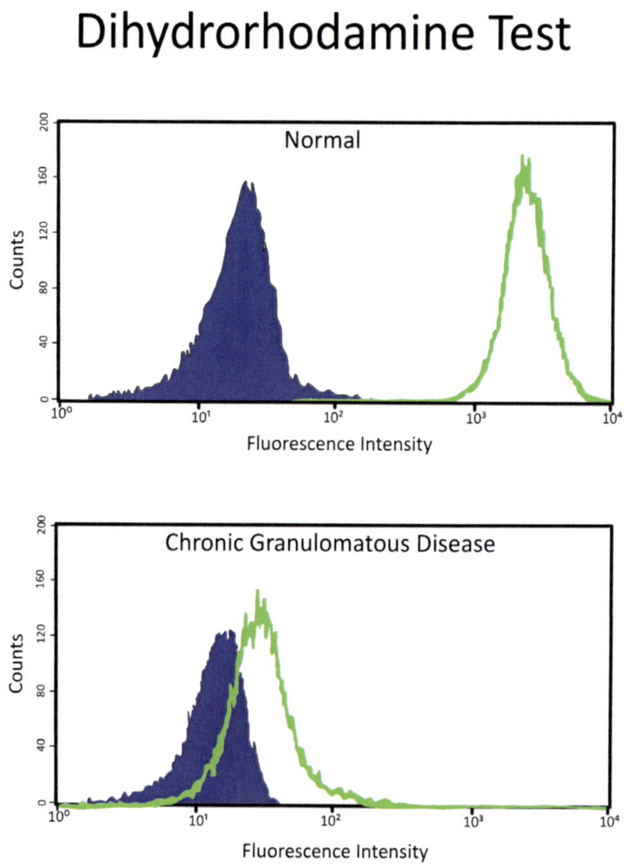

FIGURE 18.1.81 - Dihydrorhodamine Test Results

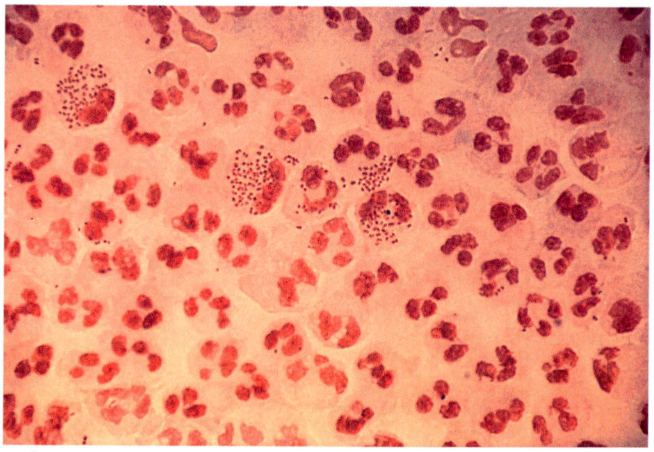

CDC/ Joe Millar, Public domain, via Wikimedia Commons

FIGURE 18.1.82 - Phagocytes Under a Gram Stain

VI. Chronic Granulomatous Disease: Management
   A. Antimicrobial prophylaxis (e.g. TMP-SMX, itraconazole)
   B. Interferon-gamma
   C. Hematopoietic stem cell transplant can be curative

VII. Myeloperoxidase Deficiency: Definition
   A. Primary immunodeficiency syndrome characterized by a defective oxidative burst within phagocytes (e.g. neutrophils, macrophages)

VIII. Myeloperoxidase Deficiency: Pathophysiology
   A. Autosomal recessive mutation in the MPO gene impairs the function of myeloperoxidase and the oxidative burst
      1. Hydrogen peroxide can no longer be converted to bleach to kill pathogens within phagocytes

IX. Myeloperoxidase Deficiency: Risk Factors
   A. Family history

X. Myeloperoxidase Deficiency: Clinical Features
   A. Majority of patients are asymptomatic
   B. Chronic *Candida albicans* infections in patients with diabetes mellitus

XI. Myeloperoxidase Deficiency: Diagnosis
   A. Flow cytometry
      1. Assesses for presence of functional myeloperoxidase
   B. Histochemical staining of leukocytes

XII. Myeloperoxidase Deficiency: Management
   A. Observation for most patients
   B. Treat infections, if they occur
   C. Caution with immunosuppressive therapies (e.g. steroids)

Immunodeficiency	Pathophysiology	Key Features	Diagnosis	Management
Chronic granulomatous disease	- Defect in NADPH oxidase - Impaired oxidative burst - X-linked recessive (more common) or autosomal recessive	- Recurrent infections with catalase-positive organisms - Granulomas can form anywhere in the body	- Dihydrorhodamine flow cytometry: diminished green fluorescence - Nitroblue tetrazolium dye test: dye remains colorless (instead of turning blue)	- Antimicrobial prophylaxis - Interferon-gamma - Hematopoietic stem cell transplant can be curative
Myeloperoxidase deficiency	- Autosomal recessive in MPO gene - Deficiency of myeloperoxidase - Impaired oxidative burst	- Most patients are asymptomatic - Chronic *Candida albicans* infections in diabetics	- Flow cytometry: absence of functional myeloperoxidase	- Observe asymptomatic patients - Treat recurrent infections, if they occur - Caution with immunosuppressive therapies

TABLE 18.1.15 - Summary of Chronic Granulomatous Disease and Myeloperoxidase Deficiency

REVIEW QUESTIONS

1. What is the pathophysiology of chronic granulomatous disease?
   - **The pathophysiology of chronic granulomatous disease can be described as an x-linked recessive defect in NADPH oxidase.**
   - **The pathophysiology of chronic granulomatous disease can be described as an impairment in the oxidative burst within phagocytes.**
   - **The pathophysiology of chronic granulomatous disease can be described as an impairment in production of superoxide, which is just another way of saying that the oxidative burst isn't working.**
   - **The pathophysiology of chronic granulomatous disease can be described as an increased susceptibility to catalase-positive organisms.**

REVIEW QUESTIONS

2. What will be the results of nitroblue tetrazolium dye test when performed on cells from patients with myeloperoxidase deficiency and on cells from patients with chronic granulomatous disease?

    - **The cells will not be able to act on the dye, and it will remain colorless.**
    - This test assesses phagocytes for the presence of NADPH oxidase. If a functional NADPH oxidase is present, the dye will turn from colorless to blue. If NADPH oxidase is absent or dysfunctional, on the other hand, the dye will remain colorless. Hence, cells from patients with myeloperoxidase deficiency will convert the dye from colorless to blue. This is in contrast to patients with chronic granulomatous disease, who have a deficiency in NADPH oxidase.
    - Patients with myeloperoxidase deficiency have a deficiency of myeloperoxidase, not NADPH oxidase.

3. A 4-year-old boy is brought to the emergency department by his mom for a "bad infection on his leg." Mom says the boy sustained a cut on his left thigh yesterday, which turned red, swollen, and painful earlier today. He has a history of two purulent skin infections caused by *Staphylococcus aureus* and a prior hospitalization for pneumonia caused by *Serratia marcescens*. The boy's maternal uncle passed away in childhood from a severe *Pseudomonas cepacia* pneumonia. Vital signs are Blood pressure 105/80 mmHg, pulse 110 beats/minute, temperature 101.3° F (38.5° C). Height and weight are in the 4th percentile. Physical examination shows a 3x3 cm purulent lesion on the boy's left thigh that is erythematous, indurated, and fluctuant. Initial laboratory evaluation shows normal leukocyte and platelet counts. Which of the following additional laboratory findings would be most consistent with this patient's clinical presentation?

    A. Giant granules within leukocytes
    B. Absence of CD18 on flow cytometry
    C. Increased green fluorescence on dihydrorhodamine flow cytometry
    D. No blue coloration following nitroblue tetrazolium dye test

- **The correct answer is option D.**
- This is a case of a 4-year-old boy with a history of recurrent cutaneous and pulmonary infections caused by catalase-positive organisms, namely *Staphylococcus aureus* and *Serratia marcescens*.
- His maternal uncle died in childhood after an infection with *Pseudomonas cepacia*, which is another catalase-positive organism.
- Because his maternal uncle was affected, the immunodeficiency in question is likely X-linked, and because the culprit organisms are all catalase-positive, the most likely underlying diagnosis is chronic granulomatous disease.
- Patients with chronic granulomatous disease suffer from recurrent infections caused by catalase-positive pathogens, such as *Staph aureus, Pseudomonas cepacia*, and *Serratia marcescens*.
- Most commonly, chronic granulomatous disease is inherited in an X-linked recessive pattern.
- Nitroblue tetrazolium dye test will not produce a blue color in patients with chronic granulomatous disease because they have a defective or deficient NADPH oxidase.
- Option A, giant granules within leukocytes, is a finding that is pathognomonic for Chediak-Higashi syndrome. Patients with Chediak-Higashi syndrome do not have a particular susceptibility to catalase-positive organisms, and they usually have pancytopenia. Since this patient's leukocyte and platelet counts were normal, Chediak-Higashi syndrome is an unlikely diagnosis.
- Option B, absence of CD18 on flow cytometry, is a finding consistent with leukocyte adhesion deficiency. This option is wrong because leukocyte adhesion deficiency is associated with infections that do not have any pus or purulence. Since this patient's lesion was purulent, leukocyte adhesion deficiency is an unlikely diagnosis.
- Option C, increased green fluorescence on dihydrorhodamine flow cytometry, is incorrect because patients with chronic granulomatous disease would have decreased green fluorescence after a dihydrorhodamine test. This is because a defective NADPH cannot convert dihydrorhodamine into rhodamine, which is the chemical responsible for the observed green fluorescence.

Pediatrics | Section 20: Congenital Phagocyte Defects - Leukocyte Adhesion Deficiency & Chediak-Higashi Syndrome

I. Leukocyte Adhesion Deficiency: Definition
   A. Primary immunodeficiency disorder characterized by the inability of leukocytes to reach the infection site

II. Leukocyte Adhesion Deficiency: Pathophysiology
   A. Autosomal recessive defect in LFA-1/CD18 component of integrins on leukocytes
   B. Neutrophils are unable to:
      1. Adhere to blood vessel walls
      2. Migrate across blood vessel walls to reach site of infection

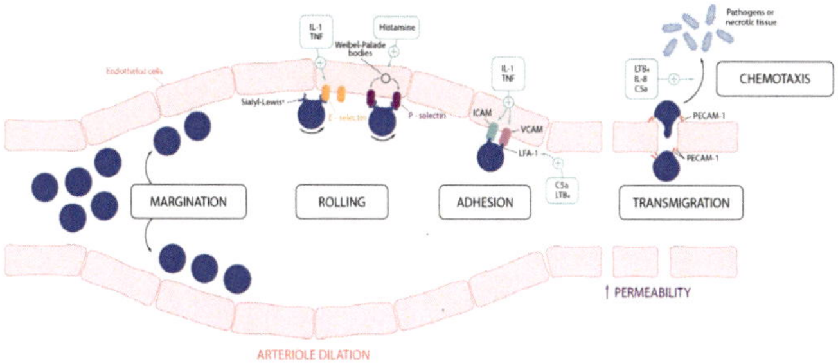

FIGURE 18.1.83 - Process of Leukocytes Traveling Within Blood Vessel to Site of Infection

III. Leukocyte Adhesion Deficiency: Risk Factors
   A. Family history

IV. Leukocyte Adhesion Deficiency: Clinical Features
   A. Recurrent bacterial infections of skin and mucosa (e.g. cellulitis, sinusitis, periodontitis)
      1. Common pathogens: *S. aureus, S. pyogenes*
      2. No pus/purulence
   B. Impaired wound healing
      1. Delayed separation of the umbilical cord stump (> 21 days)

V. Leukocyte Adhesion Deficiency: Diagnosis
   A. Laboratory evaluation
      1. Leukocytosis and neutrophilia
      2. Normal absolute lymphocyte count
   B. Biopsy of infected tissue will show no neutrophils
   C. Flow cytometry used to establish a definitive diagnosis
      1. Absence of LFA-1/CD18 on leukocytes

VI. Leukocyte Adhesion Deficiency: Management
   A. Treat recurrent infections
      1. Consider antimicrobial prophylaxis
   B. Hematopoietic stem cell transplant can be curative

VII. Chediak-Higashi Syndrome: Definition
   A. Primary immunodeficiency disorder characterized by defective lysosomal trafficking

VIII. Chediak-Higashi Syndrome: Pathophysiology
   A. Autosomal recessive mutation in the LYST gene that impairs:
      1. Lysosomal trafficking
      2. Microtubule function
   B. Lysosomes are unable to fuse with phagosomes to form phagolysosomes and kill pathogens

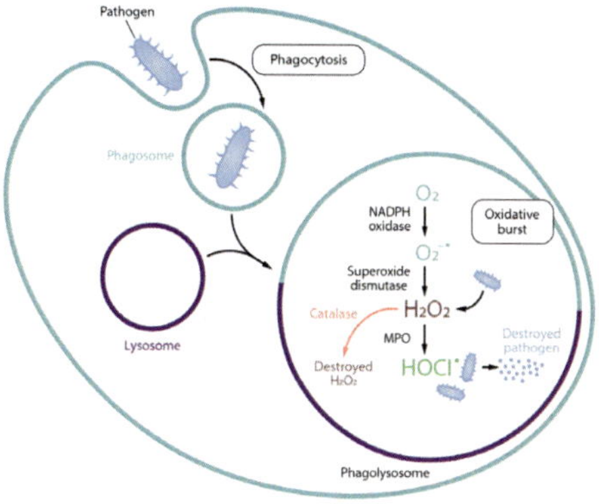

FIGURE 18.1.80 - Pathophysiology of Chronic Granulomatous Disease

IX. Chediak-Higashi Syndrome: Risk Factors
   A. Family History

X. Chediak-Higashi Syndrome: Clinical Features
   A. Recurrent infections (e.g. pneumonia, cellulitis)
      1. Common pathogens: *S. aureus* and *S. pyogenes*
   B. Partial oculocutaneous albinism
   C. Peripheral neuropathy
   D. Bleeding (e.g. epistaxis, bleeding gums)

XI. Chediak-Higashi Syndrome: Diagnosis
   A. Laboratory evaluation
      1. Pancytopenia
      2. Neutropenia
   B. Blood smear
      1. Giant azurophilic granules within leukocytes and platelets (pathognomonic finding)

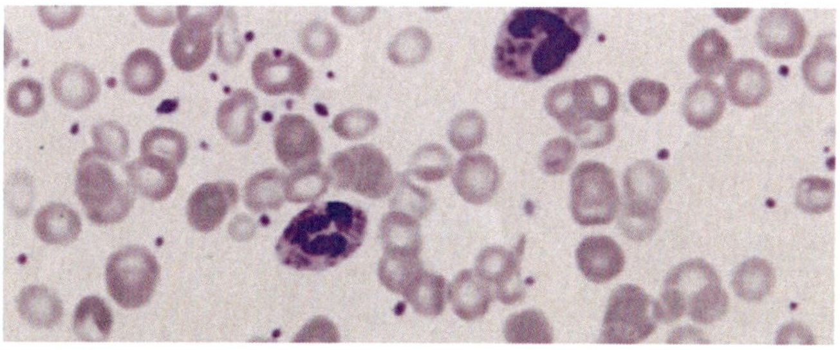

FIGURE 18.1.84 - Blood Smear of a Patient with Chediak Higashi Syndrome

XII. Chediak-Higashi Syndrome: Management
   A. Treat recurrent infections
   B. Hematopoietic stem cell transplant can be curative

Immunodeficiency	Pathophysiology	Key Features	Diagnosis	Management
Chronic granulomatous disease	- Defect in NADPH oxidase - Impaired oxidative burst - X-linked recessive (more common) or autosomal recessive	- Recurrent infections with catalase-positive organisms - Granulomas can form anywhere in the body	- Dihydrorhodamine flow cytometry: diminished green fluorescence - Nitroblue tetrazolium dye test: dye remains colorless (instead of turning blue)	- Antimicrobial prophylaxis - Interferon-gamma - Hematopoietic stem cell transplant can be curative
Myeloperoxidase deficiency	- Autosomal recessive in MPO gene - Deficiency of myeloperoxidase - Impaired oxidative burst	- Most patients are asymptomatic - Chronic *Candida albicans* infections in diabetics	- Flow cytometry: absence of functional myeloperoxidase	- Observe asymptomatic patients - Treat recurrent infections, if they occur - Caution with immunosuppressive therapies
Leukocyte adhesion deficiency	- Autosomal recessive defect in LFA-1/CD18 component of integrins on leukocytes - Leukocytes cannot adhere to or cross blood vessel walls - Leukocytes can't reach the site of infection	- Recurrent bacterial infections - No pus/purulence - Imapired wound healing - Delayed separation of umbilical cord (> 21 days)	- Flow cytometry: no LFA-1/CD18 on leukocytes - Leukocytosis, neutrophilia	- Treat recurrent infections - Hematopoietic stem cell transplant can be curative
Chediak-Higashi syndrome	- Autosomal recessive defect in LYST gene - Impaired lysosomal trafficking - Impaired formation of phagolysosomes	- Recurrent infections - Partial oculocutaneous albinism - Peripheral neuropathy - Bleeding	- Pancytopenia, especially neutropenia - Blood smear: giant azurophilic granules within leukocytes and platelets	- Treat recurrent infections - Hematopoietic stem cell transplant can be curative

TABLE 18.1.16 - Congenital Phagocyte Defects

REVIEW QUESTIONS

1. What is the key difference in the clinical presentation of soft tissue infections in patients with leukocyte adhesion deficiency compared to those otherwise healthy?

    - **The key difference is patients with leukocyte adhesion deficiency do not have any pus or purulence associated with their infections.**
    - This is because leukocytes cannot exit the blood vessels and reach the infected tissues, which means there won't be any immune cells at the site of infection to form pus. This will not be the case in otherwise healthy patients.

2. A 4-year-old boy is brought to his primary care physician by his mother for a follow-up examination after his seventh episode of Staphylococcal cellulitis. He has a history of acute otitis media and gastroenteritis. Vital signs are within normal limits. Physical examination shows white discoloration of the patient's hair and iris. Laboratory studies are significant for hemoglobin of 7 mg/dL (13.5 mg/dL - 17.5 mg/dL), white blood cell count of 2,500 cells/mm^3 (4,500 cells/mm^3 - 11,000 cells/mm^3), and a platelet count of 100,000 cells/mm^3 (150,000 cells/mm^3 - 4 00,000 cells/mm^3). The peripheral blood smear shows giant granules in neutrophils. Which of the following is the most likely underlying cause of this patient's condition?

    A. Autosomal recessive defect in LFA-1/CD18
    B. Autosomal dominant defect in LYST gene
    C. Deficient lysosomal enzyme
    D. Impaired formation of phagolysosome

    - **The correct answer is option D.**
    - This young patient presents for a follow-up visit after his seventh episode of staphylococcal cellulitis.
    - He has a history of acute otitis media and gastroenteritis. Those and numerous staph infections should raise suspicion for an immunodeficiency.
    - This patient also has albinism, evidenced by the white discoloration of the hair and iris.
    - The peripheral blood smear shows giant granules in neutrophils.
    - All these features are consistent with Chediak-Higashi syndrome.
    - Chediak-Higashi syndrome is caused by an autosomal recessive defect in the LYST gene impairing microtubule polymerization and lysosomal trafficking.
    - Functional microtubules are essential for phagolysosome formation.
    - Option A is incorrect because the autosomal recessive defect in LFA-1/CD18 protein causes leukocyte adhesion deficiency, not Chediak-Higashi syndrome.
    - Option B is incorrect because the defect in the LYST gene is autosomal recessive rather than autosomal dominant.
    - Option C is incorrect because deficient lysosomal enzymes cause lysosomal storage diseases rather than Chediak-Higashi syndrome.

Pediatrics | Section 21: Congenital Complement Deficiencies

I. Complement System Overview
   A. Proteins that form complexes to complement acute inflammation
   B. Three general complement activation pathways
      1. Classic pathway
      2. Lectin pathway
      3. Spontaneous (alternative) pathway
   C. All pathways → C3 convertase → C5 convertase → membrane attack complex (MAC)

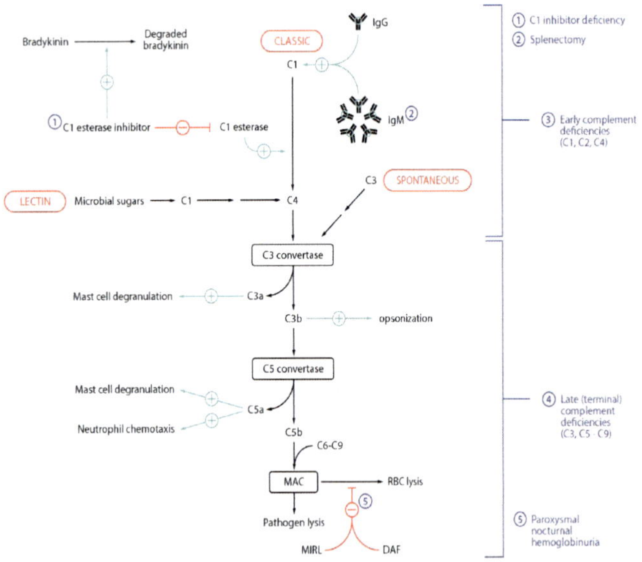

FIGURE 18.1.84 - Complement Activation Pathways

II. Hereditary Angioedema (C1 Inhibitor Deficiency): Definition
   A. Congenital disorder characterized by recurrent episodes of swelling due to a deficiency of C1 inhibitor
   B. C1 inhibitor is also known as C1 esterase inhibitor

III. Hereditary Angioedema (C1 Inhibitor Deficiency): Pathophysiology
   A. Deficiency of C1 inhibitor leads to elevated levels of bradykinin
   B. Bradykinin leads to edema via vasodilation and increased vascular permeability

IV. Hereditary Angioedema (C1 Inhibitor Deficiency): Risk Factors
   A. Family history (autosomal dominant inheritance)
   B. De novo mutations

V. Hereditary Angioedema (C1 Inhibitor Deficiency): Clinical Features
   A. Presents in late childhood or early adolescence
   B. Recurrent episodes of edema without urticaria or pruritus
      1. Common triggers: stress, trauma (e.g. dental procedures)
      2. Commonly affected areas: face, extremities, genitalia
      3. Bowel edema manifests as colicky pain, vomiting, and diarrhea
      4. Most episodes are self-limited and resolve within a few days
   C. Laryngeal edema may lead to airway compromise and death

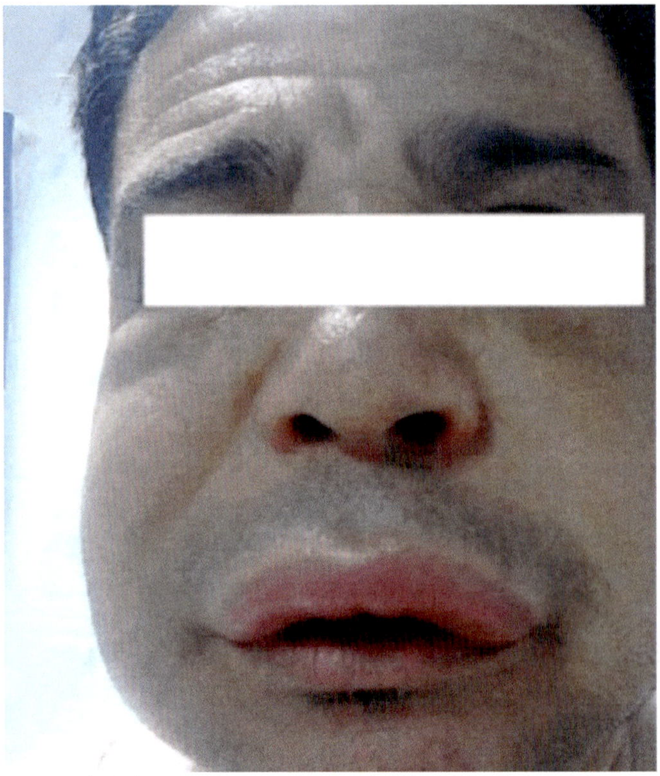

FIGURE 18.1.85 - Edema and Swelling in Hereditary Angioedema

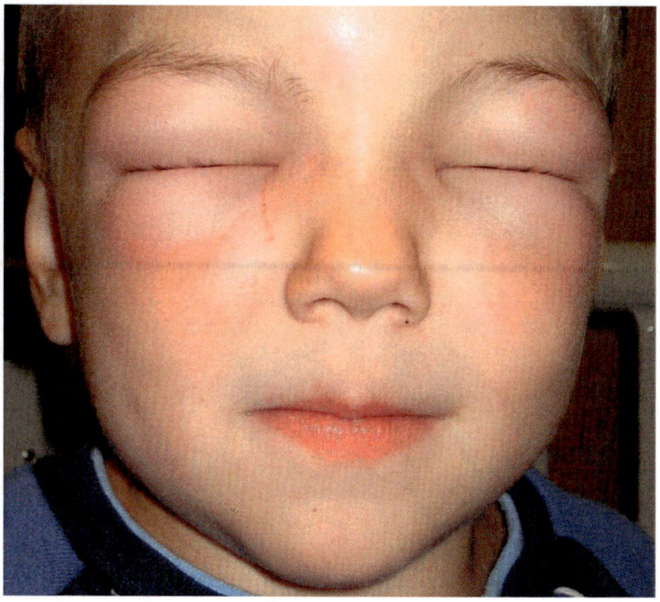

James Heilman, MD, CC BY-SA 3.0 <https://creativecommons.org/licenses/by-sa/3.0>, via Wikimedia Commons

FIGURE 18.1.86 - Edema and Swelling in Hereditary Angioedema

VI. Hereditary Angioedema (C1 Inhibitor Deficiency): Diagnosis
   A. Complement testing
      1. Low C1 inhibitor
      2. Low C4

VII. Hereditary Angioedema (C1 Inhibitor Deficiency): Management
   A. Most edema episodes are self-limited
   B. Treatment of acute edema episodes:
      1. C1 inhibitor concentrate
      2. Bradykinin antagonists (e.g. icatibant)
      3. Kallikrein inhibitors (e.g. ecallantide)
   C. FFP prior to surgeries
   D. Avoid ACE-inhibitors (e.g. lisinopril)

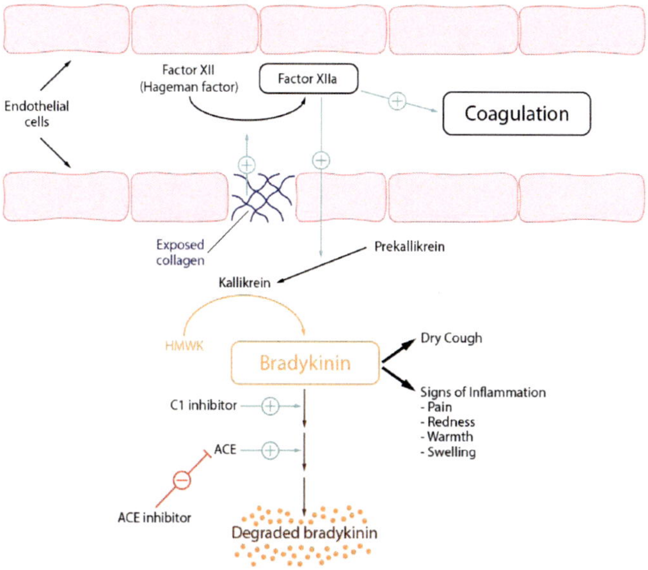

FIGURE 18.1.87 - Kinin System

VIII. Terminal Complement Deficiency (C5-C9 Deficiency): Definition
   A. An immunodeficiency disorder characterized by a deficiency of C5-C9

IX. Terminal Complement Deficiency (C5-C9 Deficiency): Pathophysiology
   A. Deficiency of C5-C9 impairs formation of the membrane attack complex (MAC)
      1. MAC kills pathogens by perforating their cell membranes

X. Terminal Complement Deficiency (C5-C9 Deficiency): Risk Factors
   A. Family history

XI. Terminal Complement Deficiency (C5-C9 Deficiency): Clinical Features
   A. Recurrent *Neisseria* infections (e.g. meningitis)
   B. Associated with lupus and glomerulonephritis

XII. Terminal Complement Deficiency (C5-C9 Deficiency): Diagnosis
   A. Complement testing
      1. Low levels of C5-C9

XIII. Terminal Complement Deficiency (C5-C9 Deficiency): Management
   A. Meningococcal vaccine
   B. Antibiotic therapy for recurrent infections

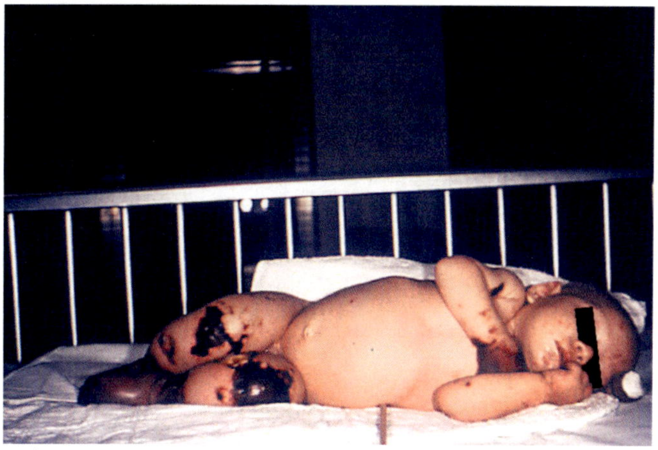

CDC/ Mr. Gust. Public domain.

FIGURE 18.1.88 - Petechiae and Purpura in Meningococcal Meningitis

REVIEW QUESTIONS

1. Facial edema that is accompanied by urticaria and/or pruritus would be more suggestive of what diagnosis?
   - **Facial edema that is accompanied by urticaria and/or pruritus should raise suspicion for anaphylaxis.**
   - The classic teaching for hereditary angioedema is that it presents with recurrent episodes of swelling that are *not* accompanied by urticaria or pruritus.

2. What is the difference between heritable angioedema and acquired angioedema?
   - **The key difference between heritable angioedema and acquired angioedema is the etiology. In heritable angioedema, bradykinin is elevated due to a congenital deficiency of C1 inhibitor. In acquired angioedema, bradykinin is elevated due to a drug-induced reaction, most commonly due to administration of ACE inhibitors.**

3. In a patient with meningitis, which unique clinical feature would be strongly suggestive of meningococcal meningitis?
   - **Petechial or purpuric rash would be strongly suggestive of meningococcal meningitis.**
   - Clinicians should suspect meningococcal meningitis when patients have a petechial or a purpuric rash on their body, especially on the lower extremities, in addition to all other clinical features of meningitis, such as neck stiffness or altered mental status.

4. A 14-year-old girl is brought to the emergency department by her mom. She says she took her daughter to the dentist this morning, and a few minutes into the procedure, her daughter's face started to swell up. The swelling got progressively worse, which prompted their visit to the hospital. On review of systems, the girl endorses colicky abdominal pain and denies itching. Vital signs include blood pressure 110/75 mmHg, pulse 71 beats/minute, and temperature 97.2° F (36.2° C). Physical examination shows significant periorbital swelling as well as swelling of the upper lip. Cardiopulmonary examination is unremarkable, and there are no rashes or scratch marks. Which of the following is the most likely cause of this patient's condition?

   A. IgE-mediated allergic reaction
   B. Impaired degradation of bradykinin
   C. Type IV hypersensitivity
   D. C5-C9 deficiency

- **The correct answer is option B.**
- This is a case of a 14-year-old girl who developed facial swelling during a dental procedure that got progressively worse.
- Her swelling was accompanied by colicky abdominal pain, but no itching and no rashes.
- Her physical examination shows significant periorbital swelling and swelling of the upper lip.
- In the setting of normal vital signs and an unremarkable cardiopulmonary examination, this presentation is strongly suggestive of hereditary angioedema.
- Hereditary angioedema typically presents in late childhood or early adolescence, and it often follows trauma, for example during dental procedures. The episodes of edema are not accompanied by urticaria or pruritus. Also, patients may present with colicky abdominal pain due to bowel edema, which is the likely explanation of this patient's colicky abdominal pain.
- Hereditary angioedema is characterized by a deficiency of C1 esterase inhibitor, which impairs degradation of bradykinin and thus leads to elevated levels of bradykinin.
- Option A, IgE-mediated allergic reaction, is incorrect because that would be a plausible etiology of anaphylaxis. Since our patient's facial swelling was not accompanied by itching, rashes, or cardiopulmonary compromise, anaphylaxis is unlikely.
- Option C is incorrect because type IV hypersensitivity is a common etiology of rashes due to skin contact with poison ivy or nickel. This patient has no rashes on physical examination.
- Option D is incorrect because deficiency of C5 through C9 does not lead to edema. Rather, these patients usually present with recurrent *Neisseria* infections.

Pediatrics | Section 22: Juvenile Idiopathic Arthritis

I. General Information
   A. The most common chronic rheumatic disease of childhood that manifest before the age of 16
   B. Usually affects girls > boys
   C. Most commonly idiopathic etiology
   D. HLA association

II. Pathophysiology
   A. Multifactorial: genetic and environmental factors → autoimmune mechanism → inflammation of synovium with infiltration of inflammatory cells that can eventually result in decreased or function loss

III. Clinical Features
   A. Articular: joint pain, stiffness, swelling, erythema
   B. Generalized fatigue
   C. Fever
   D. Rash
   E. Hepatosplenomegaly
   F. Blurry, dry, painful, red eyes; photophobia (anterior uveitis)
   G. Complications:
      1. Macrophage activation syndrome (MAS): systemic JIA
      2. Blindness, glaucoma: anterior uveitis
      3. Leg length discrepancy, limited joint mobility, joint destruction, ↓ growth

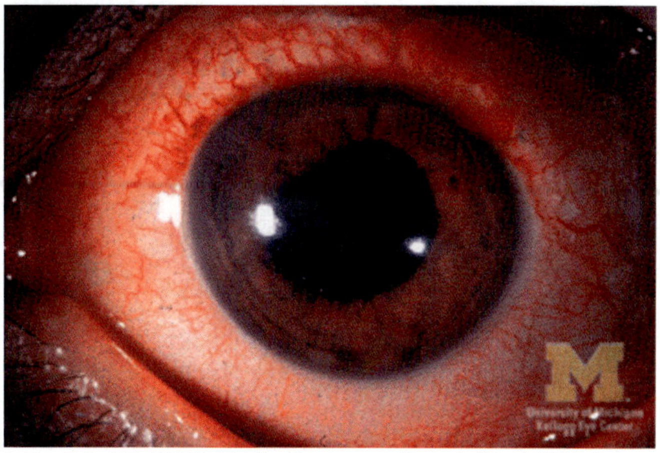

FIGURE 18.1.90 - Anterior Uveitis

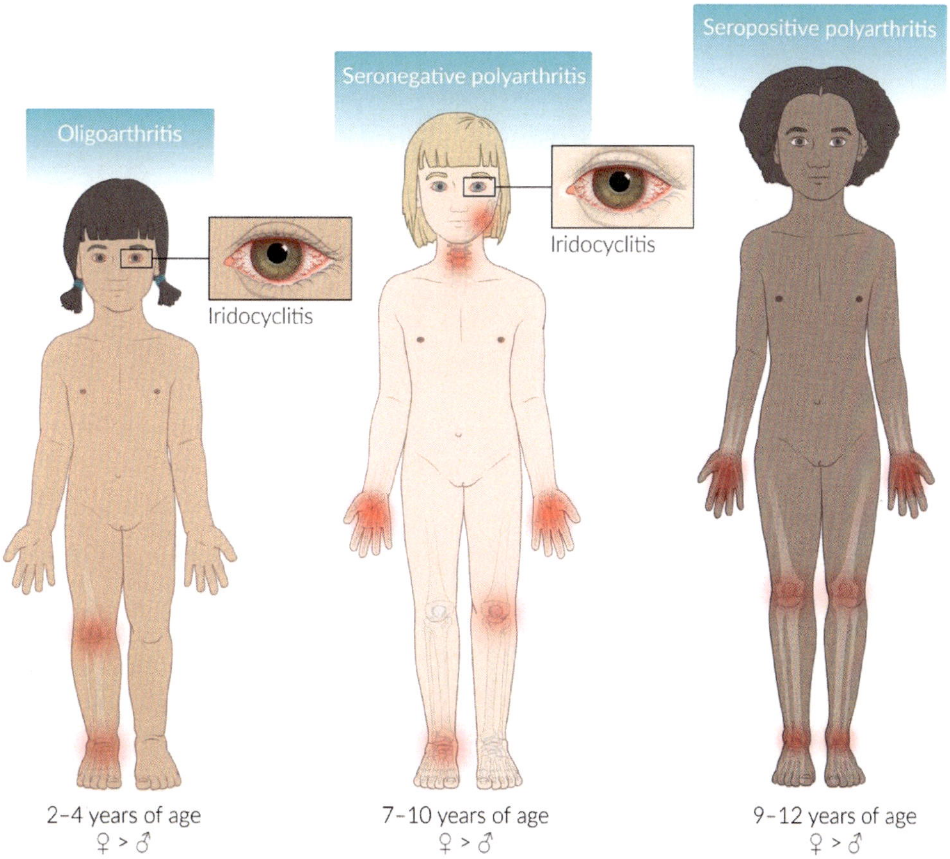

FIGURE 18.1.89 - Different Types of Juvenile Idiopathic Arthritis

	Oligoarticular JIA	Seronegative polyarticular JIA	Seropositive polyarticular JIA	Systemic JIA
Definition	- Arthritis affecting ≤ 4 joints in the first 6 months of the disease - Also called "pauci-arthritis"	- Arthritis involving ≥ 5 joints in the first 6 months of the disease		- Arthritis + intermittent fever ≥ 2 weeks + at least one of the extra-articular manifestations - Also called "Still disease"
General information	- Most common form - Girls > boys - Peak incidence 2-4 years	- Girls > boys - Bimodal distribution: 2-4 and 6-12	- Girls > boys - Late childhood to adolescence	- Girls = boys - Peak incidence 2-4 years
Articular manifestations	- Asymmetrical involvement - Weight-bearing joints: knees and ankles (not hips)	- Symmetrical/asymmetrical - Small and large joints: metacarpal-phalangeal joints, the wrist, temporomandibular joint, cervical spine	- Symmetrical - Smaller joints: interphalangeal joints	- ≥ 2 joints
Extra-articular manifestations	- Anterior uveitis	- Anterior uveitis	- Subcutaneous nodules	- Salmon-colored rash, generalized lymphadenopathy, hepatosplenomegaly, serositis
Diagnosis/ Laboratory findings	- ↑ ESR, + ANA, - RF - Slit-lamp (uveitis)	- ↑ ESR, + ANA, - RF - Slit-lamp (uveitis)	- ↑ ESR, + RF	- ↑ ESR, - RF - No autoantibodies - Anemia, thrombocytosis, leukocytosis
Management	- NSAIDs (e.g. ibuprofen) - Steroids: intraarticular, eye drops - DMARDs (e.g. methotrexate)	- NSAIDs - DMARDs (e.g. methotrexate)		- NSAIDs - Steroids - Tocilizumab (IL-6 inhibitor)

TABLE 18.1.17 - Juvenile Idiopathic Arthritis

Systemic juvenile idiopathic arthritis (Still disease)

Etiology
Idiopathic

Epidemiology
♀ = ♂
Peak age of onset: 2–4 years

Serology
Typically negative for autoantibodies

Laboratory studies
Anemia, leukocytosis, thrombocytosis

Complications
Macrophage activation syndrome (MAS)

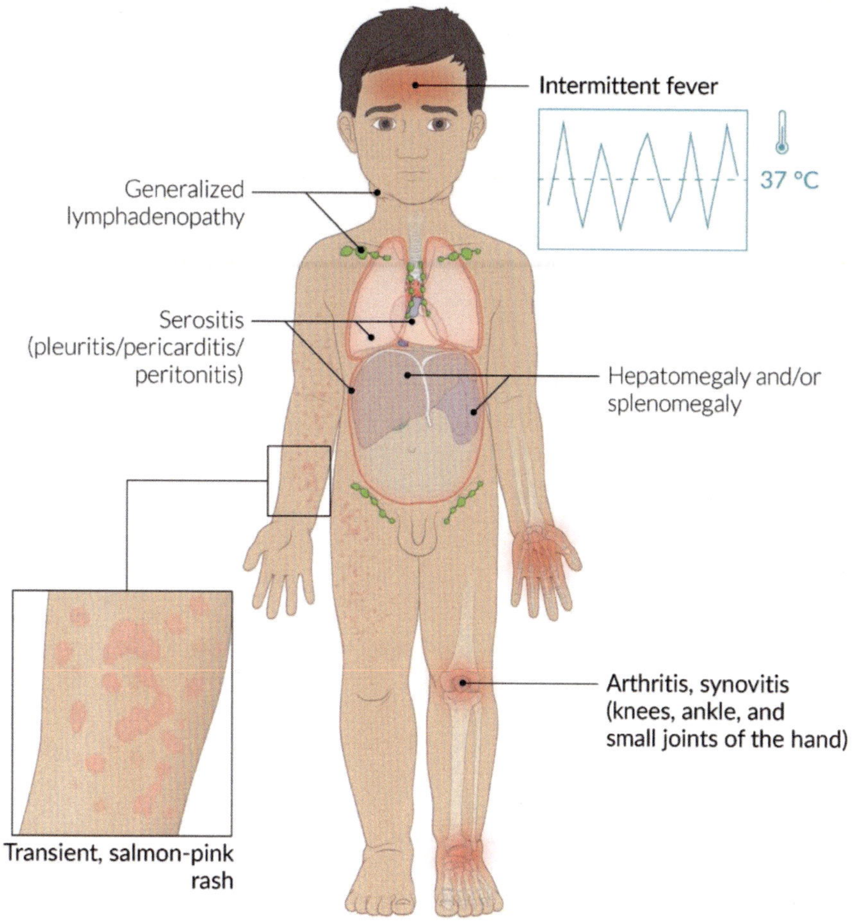

FIGURE 18.1.91 - Child with Systemic Juvenile Idiopathic Arthritis

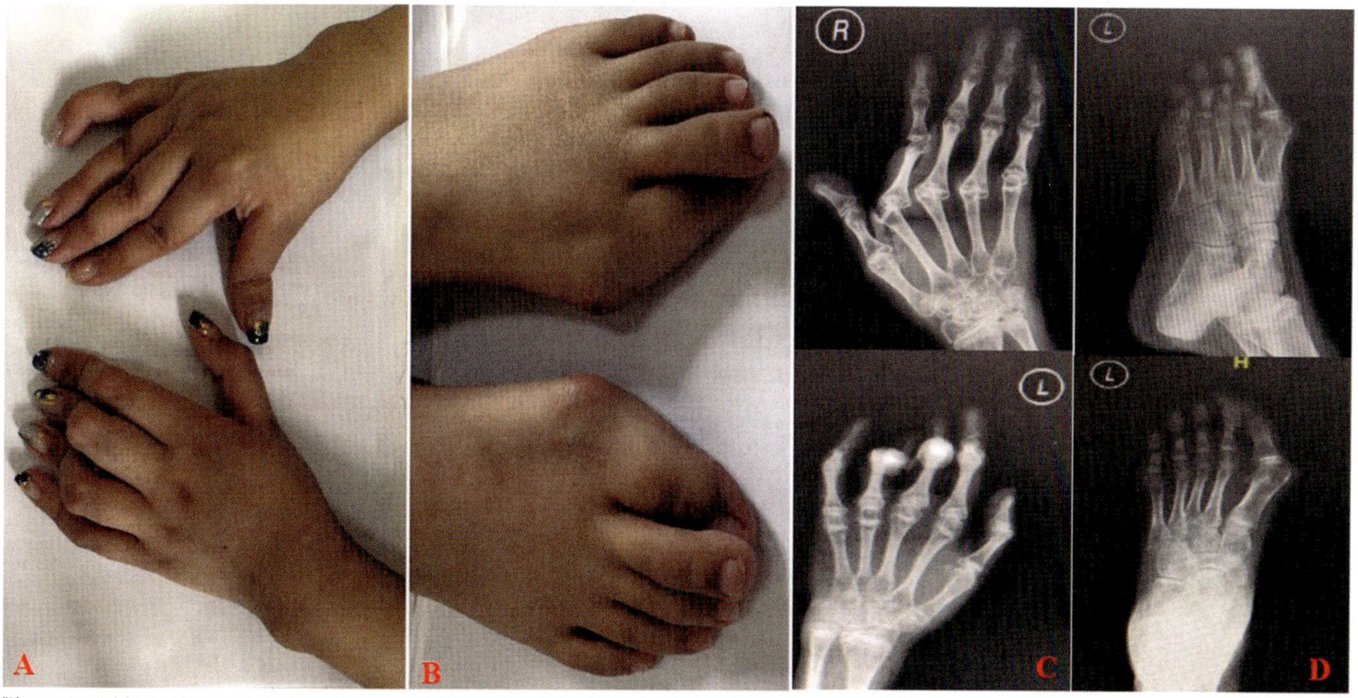

FIGURE 18.1.92 - Patient with Swollen Metatarsal & Interphalangeal Joints

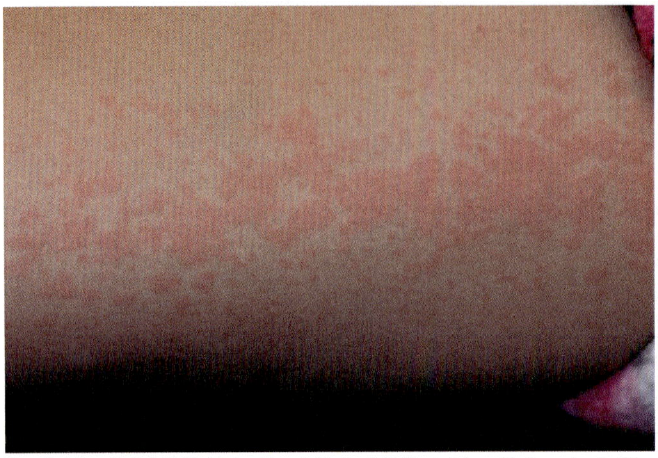

FIGURE 18.1.93 - Salmon-Colored Rash

IV. Diagnosis
   A. Diagnostic criteria:
      1. Disease onset <16 years
      2. Arthritis lasting for more than 6 weeks
   B. Laboratory: inflammatory markers, CBC, autoantibodies
   C. Ophthalmological examination: slit lamp exam
      1. Every 3 months for detection of uveitis in high risk patients
      2. Every 12 months for everyone else

V. Management
   A. Medications
      1. NSAIDs + intra-articular steroids: first line
      2. DMARDs, systemic glucocorticoids, biological agents: second-line
   B. Supportive treatment
      1. Exercises to improve mobility, surgery, orthotics
   C. Slit lamp exam every 1-3 months to monitor response to treatment in patients with anterior uveitis

VI. Prognosis
   A. Mostly resolve by puberty
   B. Poor prognosis
      1. Positive family history of the disease,
      2. Early disease onset: higher level of impairment
      3. Higher number of affected joints at onset of disease
      4. Rheumatoid factor (RF) positive, anti CCP-antibodies positive

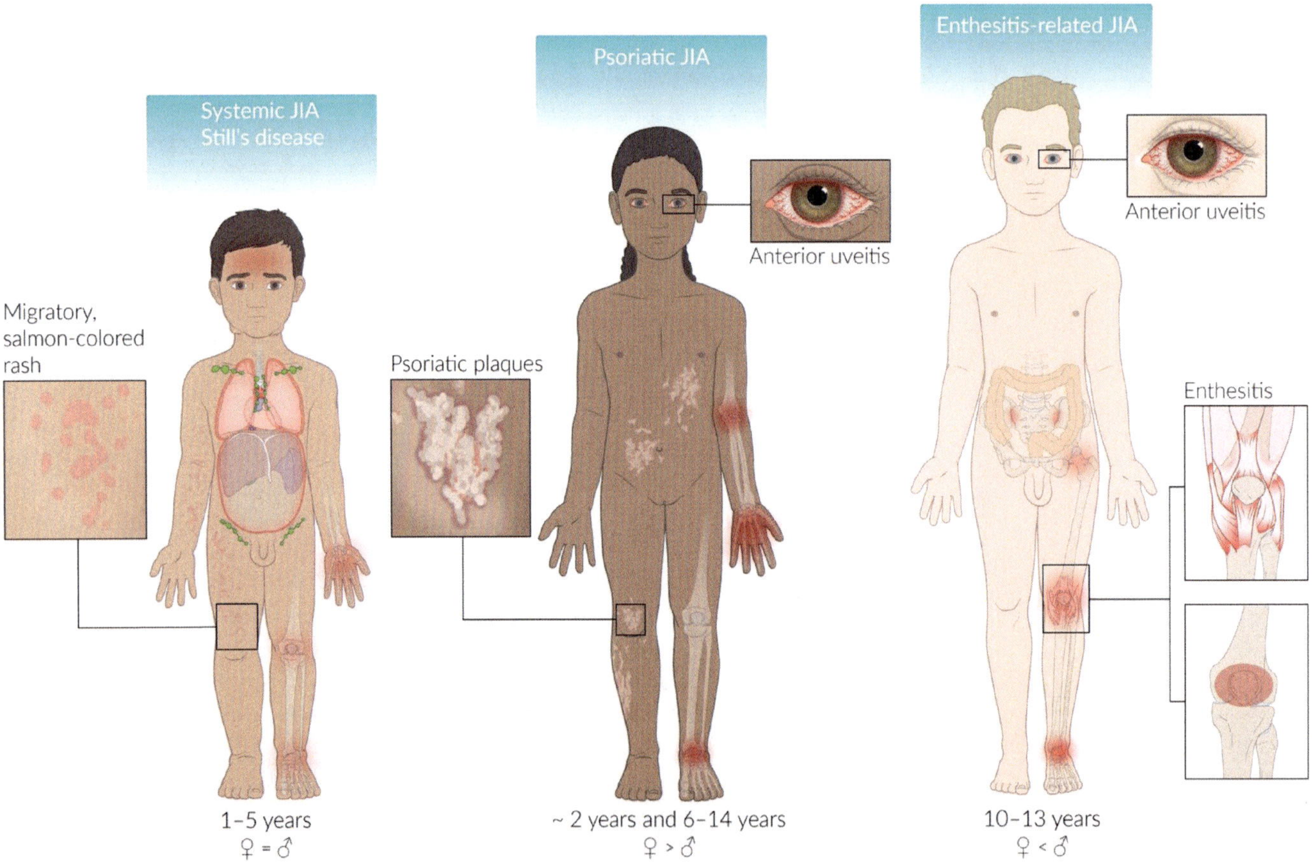

FIGURE 18.1.94 - Less Common Types of Juvenile Idiopathic Arthritis

REVIEW QUESTIONS

1. A 2-year-old girl is brought to the physician due to recurrent episodes of pain and swelling in her right knee and ankle for 3 months. Her parents also notice her activity level has decreased and she appears tired more frequently. She attends daycare and has not had any trauma. Joint examination reveals tenderness, mild swelling, and erythema of the right knee and ankle joints. The rest of the examination is normal. Laboratory results show an elevated ESR, positive ANA, and negative rheumatoid factor. What is the most likely diagnosis of this patient?
    - **The most likely diagnosis of this patient would be Oligoarthritis JIA**
    - This 2-year-old girl is presenting with recurrent episodes of pain and swelling in her right knee and ankle as well as tiredness for 3 months.
    - Laboratory results reveal elevated inflammatory markers such as ESR.
    - Chronic arthritis in a patient <16 years old is highly suggestive of juvenile idiopathic arthritis.
    - The asymmetrical distribution of major joints such as the knee and ankle joints, the positive ANA, and the negative rheumatoid factor all support the diagnosis of oligoarthritis subtype of JIA.
    - Oligoarthritis JIA affects ≤ 4 joints in the first 6 months of the disease and girls are more commonly affected than boys.

2. A 10-year-old girl is brought to the physician by her parents due to recurrent episodes of fever and joint pain. She has had pain in her knees, her hands, and her ankles bilaterally for the past 4 months. Her parents have associated it with "growing pains", but the pain has not improved. Physical exam reveals tenderness, swelling, and erythema involving the metacarpophalangeal joints, knees, and ankles bilaterally. Subcutaneous nodules can be seen on the extensor surfaces of both elbows. Laboratory evaluations show an ESR of 50 mm/h (N=0-20 mm/h). On further evaluation, which of the following will likely be present in this patient?

    A. Chronic anterior uveitis
    B. Generalized lymphadenopathy
    C. Positive rheumatoid factor
    D. Hepatosplenomegaly

- **The correct answer is C.**
- This 10-year-old patient is presenting with arthritis for 4 months.
- Her hands, knees, and ankles are involved bilaterally and are tender, swollen, and erythematous on physical exam.
- The ESR is also elevated.
- Chronic arthritis and fever manifesting in patients < 16 years make juvenile idiopathic arthritis the most likely diagnosis.
- Her age, the symmetrical involvement of joints, as well as the subcutaneous nodules on the extensor surfaces of both elbows make seropositive polyarticular JIA the most likely diagnosis.
- Patients with seropositive polyarticular JIA are typically positive for rheumatoid factor, so the correct choice is option C.
- Recall that in seropositive polyarticular JIA, joints are symmetrically involved and smaller joints such as the interphalangeal joints are commonly affected like we see in our patient.Large joints such as knees and ankles may also be affected.
- Also, patients may have subcutaneous nodules on the extensor surfaces of elbows and the Achilles tendon.
- Again, the patient has all of these classic features.
- Option A is incorrect because chronic anterior uveitis is not associated with seropositive polyarticular JIA.
- Instead, it's most commonly associated with oligoarthritis and seronegative polyarticular JIA among others.
- Options B and D are incorrect because patients with systemic JIA or Still's disease present with generalized lymphadenopathy and hepatosplenomegaly, not patients with seropositive polyarticular JIA.

Pediatrics | Section 23: Epiglottitis and Croup

I. Epiglottitis: General Characteristics
   A. Inflammation of the epiglottis and surrounding supraglottis
   B. Previously due to *Haemophilus influenzae* type b (Hib)
      1. Rare with widespread immunization
      2. Keep Hib on the differential in unvaccinated children
      3. Other etiologies: *Streptococcus pyogenes, Streptococcus pneumoniae, Staphylococcus aureus*
   C. More common in young children but can occur in unimmunized adults

II. Epiglottitis: Clinical Features
   A. Acute high fever, sore throat, anxiety
   B. Dysphagia, odynophagia, drooling, muffled "hot-potato" voice
   C. Tripod position: patient leans forward and extends the neck, increasing the airway diameter to ease their breathing
   D. Signs of respiratory distress: retractions, cyanosis, inspiratory stridor

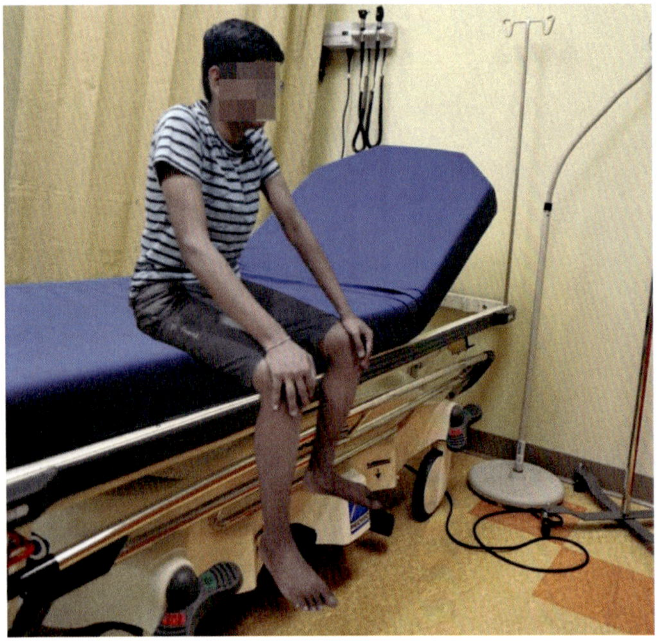

FIGURE 18.1.95 - Tripod Positioning

III. Epiglottitis: Diagnosis
   A. Clinical diagnosis
   B. Labs: CBC, blood culture, epiglottal culture if intubated
      1. Avoid drawing labs until the airway is stable due to the risk of respiratory distress and obstruction with agitation
   C. Diagnostic laryngoscopy: "cherry-red" epiglottis
   D. Soft tissue lateral neck X-ray: "thumbprint sign"
      1. Enlarged epiglottis with supraglottic narrowing

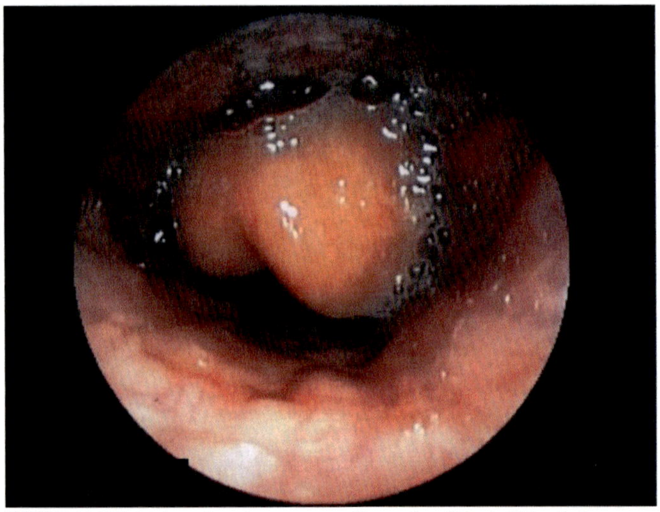

FIGURE 18.1.96 - Laryngoscopy: "Cherry-Red" Epiglottis

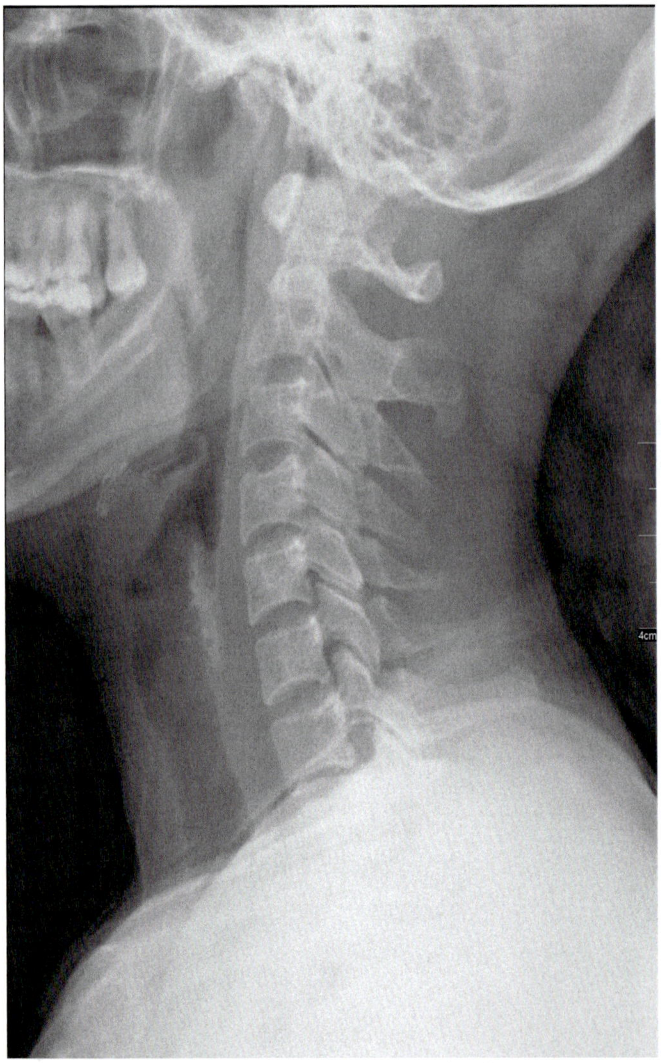

FIGURE 18.1.97 - Lateral Neck X-ray of a Healthy Person

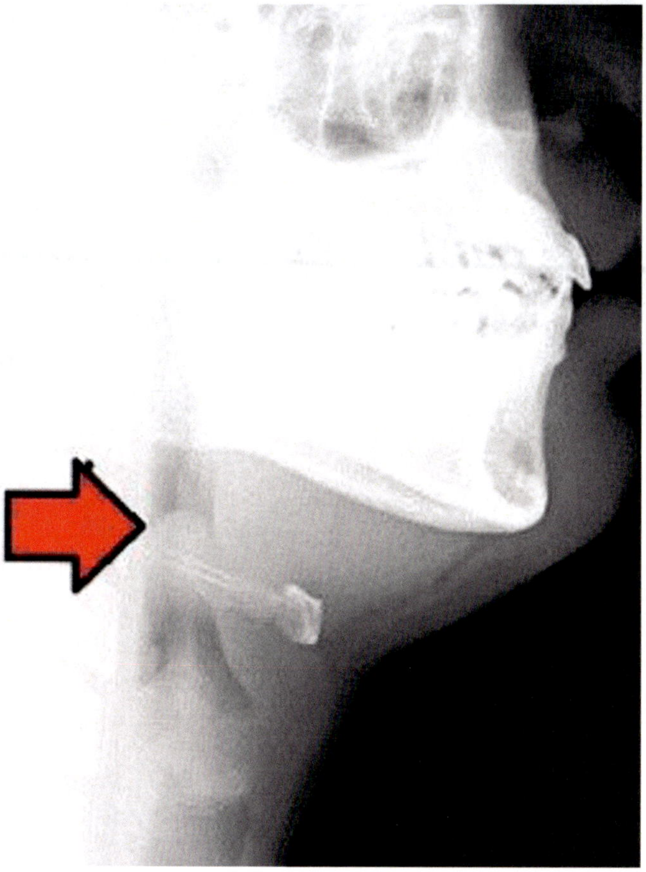

FIGURE 18.1.98 - Lateral Neck X-ray: "Thumbprint Sign" in Epiglottitis

IV. Epiglottitis: Management
  A. Airway management
    1. Keep the patient comfortable and calm
    2. Supplemental oxygen
    3. Evaluate for signs of impending airway obstruction such as stridor, tachypnea, retractions, altered mental status
    4. Bag-valve ventilation with 100% oxygen
    5. Intubate if needed
  B. Empiric antibiotics
    1. Choose antibiotic active against Hib and the other common causes of epiglottitis
    2. Third-generation cephalosporin and vancomycin
  C. If patient has Hib, post-exposure prophylaxis of close contacts with rifampin
    1. Important for unvaccinated children and the immunocompromised

V. Croup: General Characteristics
  A. Also known as laryngotracheitis
  B. Inflammation of the larynx and subglottic airway
  C. Most commonly due to viruses
    1. Parainfluenza most common
    2. Others: RSV, coronaviruses, adenoviruses, enteroviruses
  D. Most common ages 6 months to 3 years
  E. Most common in fall and winter months

VI. Croup: Clinical Features
  A. Rhinorrhea, congestion, fever, hoarseness
  B. "Seal-bark" cough that may eventually lead to stridor
  C. In severe disease, patient may have stridor at rest, hypoxemia, and respiratory distress
  D. Always watch for signs of impending respiratory failure
    1. Lethargy, severe retractions, decreased level of consciousness, tachycardia, cyanosis

VII. Croup: Diagnosis
  A. Clinical diagnosis
  B. Laboratory testing typically not required
  C. Chest X-ray not required, but may show "steeple sign" due to subglottic narrowing

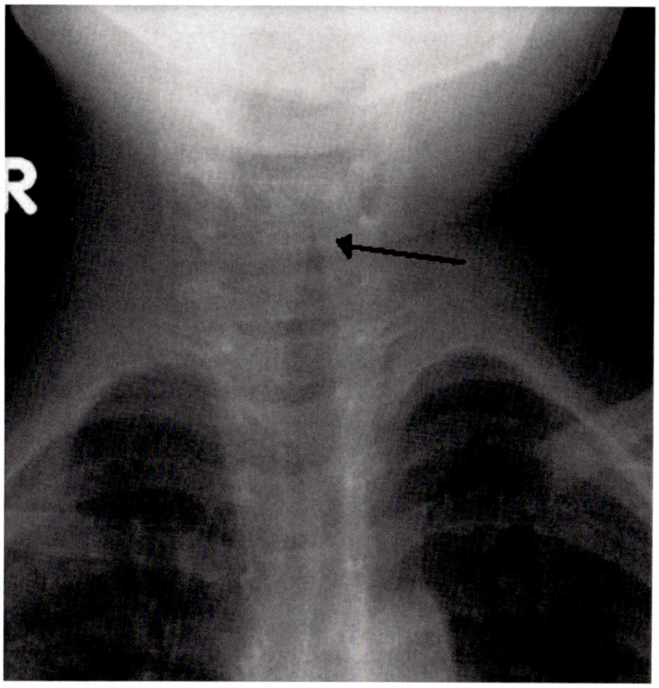

FIGURE 18.1.99 - Chest X-ray: "Steeple Sign" in Croup

VIII. Croup: Management
  A. Mild croup (no stridor at rest)
    1. Supportive care
    2. Single-dose of oral dexamethasone
  B. Moderate/severe croup (stridor at rest)
    1. Supportive care, humidified oxygen
    2. Dexamethasone
    3. Racemic epinephrine
  C. Indications for hospitalization
    1. Severe symptoms after initial treatment
    2. Altered level of consciousness
    3. Impending respiratory failure
    4. Supplemental oxygen requirement
    5. Severe dehydration

Condition	Etiology	Key Features
Epiglottitis	- Inflammation of epiglottis and surrounding supraglottis - Most commonly bacterial infection	- Drooling, dysphagia, muffled voice - Tripod position - "Thumbprint" sign on lateral neck X-ray
Croup	- Inflammation of larynx and subglottic airway - Most commonly due to parainfluenza virus	- "Seal-bark" cough - Inspiratory stridor - "Steeple sign" on chest X-ray

TABLE 18.1.18 - Epiglottitis and Croup

REVIEW QUESTIONS

1. A 7-year-old boy is brought to the emergency department by his mother because of fever and difficulty breathing for the past 2 hours. He suddenly felt sick today, and his breathing has worsened since the onset of symptoms. He is not vaccinated due to parental preferences. Physical examination shows he is distressed sitting in his mother's lap, leaning forward, and extending his neck. Stridor is audible, and he is using accessory muscles to breathe. His vital signs show he is febrile, tachypnic and hypoxic to 85%. What is the best next step in management?
   - **The best next step in management is bag-valve-mask and 100% oxygen. Intubation should be considered if he is not protecting his airways or tiring out.**
   - This boy presents with a sudden onset of fever and difficulty breathing. He is in acute hypoxic respiratory failure.
   - He is sitting in his mother's lap, leaning forward, and extending his neck. This is called a tripod position, which helps with supraglottic obstruction to widen the airways.
   - Considering that this patient is not vaccinated, all of the above findings are concerning for acute epiglottitis.
   - Given this boy is unstable and in acute distress, the first thing to do is assess the ABCs. Assisted ventilation can be started with bag-valve-mask and 100% oxygen, with a transition to intubation if needed.

2. A 3-year-old girl is brought to her primary care physician by her parents due to a severe cough that started 2 days ago. Her parents have also noticed a runny nose and mild fever for the past week. Physical examination shows a somnolent girl with a high-pitched, grunting sound on inspiration and episodes of cough. What is the strongest indication for hospitalization?
   - **The strongest indication for hospitalization is somnolence.**
   - This girl presents with a severe cough, runny nose, and mild fever.
   - She also has a high-pitched, grunting sound on inspiration, most consistent with stridor.
   - Given all these findings, the most likely diagnosis is croup.
   - The fact that she is somnolent indicates severe upper airway obstruction and possible hypoxemia, causing altered mental status. Somnolence is the strongest indication for hospitalization of this particular patient.

Pediatrics | Section 24: Bacterial Tracheitis, Pertussis, and Bronchiolitis

I. Bacterial Tracheitis: General Characteristics
   A. Invasive exudative bacterial infection of the soft tissues of the trachea
   B. Usually in the setting of previous airway mucosal damage from a viral infection
   C. More common in young children
   D. More common in the fall and winter
   E. Most common pathogens: *Staphylococcus aureus, Streptococcus pneumoniae, Streptococcus pyogenes, Moraxella catarrhalis*

II. Bacterial Tracheitis: Clinical Features
   A. Signs and symptoms of viral respiratory tract infection one to three days before more severe respiratory illness
   B. Signs of airway obstruction: stridor, cough, respiratory distress
   C. May be associated with odynophagia or dysphagia

III. Bacterial Tracheitis: Diagnosis
   A. May appear to have croup, but responds poorly to racemic epinephrine
   B. Imaging and laboratory findings are nonspecific
      1. Chest X-ray reveals "steeple-sign" and irregularity of the tracheal wall
      2. Order cultures and viral testing of respiratory specimens
   C. Definitive diagnosis requires direct visualization of the airway
      1. Reveals adherent mucopurulent membranes in the trachea

IV. Bacterial Tracheitis: Management
   A. Airway management
      1. Determine the severity of airway obstruction and intubate if needed
   B. Supportive care
      1. Supplemental oxygen, IV fluids, trial of racemic epinephrine
   C. Empiric antibiotics
      1. Vancomycin plus a third-generation cephalosporin

V. Pertussis: General Characteristics
   A. Also known as "whooping cough"
   B. Bordetella pertussis
      1. Pertussis toxin: causes systemic manifestations such as hypoglycemia, lymphocytosis
   C. Most common in children < 1 year of age
   D. More common in the summer and fall
   E. Transmitted through respiratory droplets; highly contagious

VI. Pertussis: Clinical Features
   A. Three stages of infection
   B. Catarrhal stage (1 - 2 weeks)
      1. Nonspecific upper respiratory symptoms such as cough, nasal discharge
      2. Cough will gradually worsen
      3. Most contagious in this stage
   C. Paroxysmal stage (2 - 8 weeks)
      1. Paroxysmal coughing followed by high pitched whooping sound
      2. Cough may have tongue protrusion, gagging, cyanosis
      3. May have posttussive vomiting
      4. Infants may not have the characteristic cough
   D. Convalescent stage (weeks to months after initial infection)
      1. Gradual reduction in symptoms
      2. May continue to have coughing attacks

VII. Pertussis: Diagnosis
   A. Clinical diagnosis
   B. Lab findings
      1. CBC may show lymphocyte-predominant leukocytosis
      2. Culture or PCR is gold-standard for diagnosis

VIII. Pertussis: Management
   A. Antibiotics
      1. > 1 month of age: any macrolide
      2. < 1 month of age: azithromycin
   B. Hospitalization
      1. Infants < 4 months, respiratory distress, cyanosis, apnea
      2. Supportive care
   C. Post-exposure prophylaxis
      1. Macrolides
      2. Household and close contacts
      3. Required even if immunized

IX. Bronchiolitis: General Characteristics
   A. Lower airway viral infection that is most common in children < 2 years of age
   B. More common in the winter months
   C. Common etiologies include respiratory syncytial virus, rhinovirus, influenza, parainfluenza virus, adenoviruses, coronaviruses
   D. Risk factors for increased severity: prematurity, cardiac disease, chronic pulmonary disease, smokers in the home, daycare attendance

X. Bronchiolitis: Clinical Features
   A. Preceding upper respiratory symptoms: rhinorrhea, congestion
   B. Fever, cough, and signs of respiratory distress
      1. Retractions, head bobbing, nasal flaring, grunting, tachypnea, apnea, cyanosis
   C. Auscultation may reveal wheezing, rales, or rhonchi
   D. Signs of dehydration: decreased capillary refill, dry mucous membranes, tachycardia, sunken fontanelles

XI. Bronchiolitis: Diagnosis
   A. Can be difficult to distinguish from pneumonia
   B. Laboratory testing generally not required
   C. Chest X-ray is not required
      1. Findings include peribronchial thickening, hyperinflation, atelectasis, patchy and scattered infiltrate

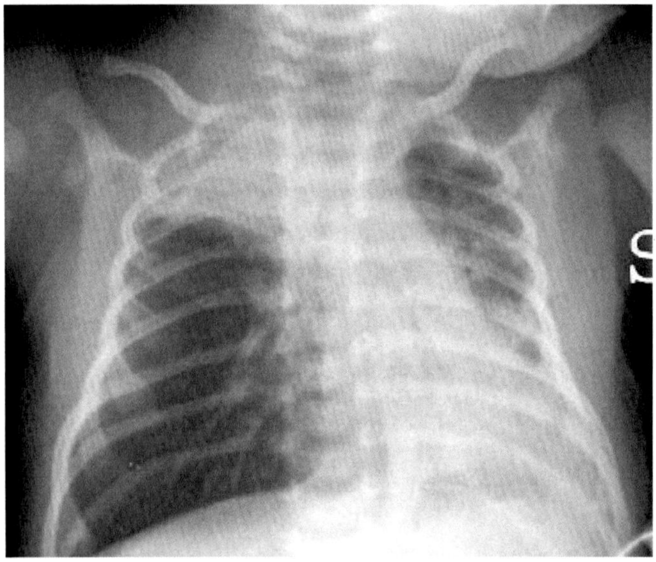

FIGURE 18.1.100 - Chest X-Ray: Hyperinflation and Areas of Atelectasis in Bronchiolitis

XII. Bronchiolitis: Management
   A. Respiratory support
      1. In children with persistent desaturations, use supplemental oxygen
      2. May require CPAP or endotracheal intubation if severe
   B. Most medications have little to no benefit
   C. Monitor hydration status
      1. Administer IV fluids if patient has poor oral intake
   D. Indications for hospitalization
      1. Toxic appearance, poor feeding, dehydration
      2. Worsening respiratory distress or impending respiratory failure
   E. Prevention
      1. High-risk infants (premature, congenital heart disease, pulmonary disease) may receive palivizumab
      2. Monoclonal antibody against RSV

REVIEW QUESTIONS

1. A 5-year-old boy is brought to the hospital for difficulty breathing for the past 2 hours. He was admitted 5 days ago with stridor, runny nose, and mild fever. Racemic epinephrine and inhaled dexamethasone were administered for presumed croup. Vital signs are significant for a temperature of 102.2° F (39° C). His arterial oxygen saturation is 92%. Physical exam shows persistent stridor. What is the best next step in confirming this patients diagnosis?

   - **The diagnostic modality used to diagnose this patient's current condition is bronchoscopy and laryngoscopy.**
   - This patient presents with difficulty breathing, stridor, and fever.
   - He initially was administered racemic epinephrine and inhaled dexamethasone for presumed croup. However, his condition has not improved.
   - Therefore, this patient most likely has bacterial tracheitis, which does not respond to the typical management of croup.
   - The diagnosis of bacterial tracheitis can be confirmed with bronchoscopy and laryngoscopy, which reveal adherent mucopurulent membranes.

2. A 1-day-old girl is evaluated in the hospital. She was born at 35 weeks of gestation via vaginal delivery. Apgar scores were 6 and 7 at 1 and 5 minutes, respectively. A murmur was heard at the mid-left sternal border several hours after birth. An echocardiogram shows a narrow pulmonary infundibulum, right ventricular hypertrophy, a ventricular septal defect, and an overriding aorta. Chest X-ray shows clear lungs. What is the strongest indication for this patient to receive prophylactic palivizumab against bronchiolitis?

   - **The strongest indication for this patient to receive prophylactic palivizumab against bronchitis is tetralogy of Fallot.**
   - This baby girl was born at 35 weeks of gestation, a late preterm period.
   - She had a murmur auscultated several hours after birth with Echo findings of tetralogy of fallout.
   - Chest X-ray showed clear lungs.
   - High-risk (i.e. prematurity, congenital heart disease, lung disease) patients should receive the prophylactic vaccination.

Pediatrics | Section 25: Pneumonia

I. Pediatric Pneumonia: General Characteristics
   A. Inflammatory condition of lungs involving the lung parenchyma
   B. First month of life: GBS or gram-negative enteric bacilli
   C. Younger than five years: Most often viral
   D. Community-acquired
      1. *Streptococcus pneumoniae* most common
      2. Staphylococcus aureus
      3. Moraxella catarrhalis
   E. Atypical pneumonia: *Mycoplasma pneumoniae and Chlamydophila pneumoniae*
   F. Typical bacterial pathogens usually cause lobar pneumonia
   G. Viral and atypicals usually cause bronchiolitis or interstitial pneumonitis

II. Pediatric Pneumonia: Clinical Features
   A. Neonates and infants
      1. Fever, lethargy
      2. May have history of apnea
   B. Older children
      1. Fever, cough, increased work of breathing
   C. Physical exam
      1. Tachypnea, cough, fever
      2. Severe cases may be associated with hypoxia and respiratory failure
      3. Auscultation may reveal rales, wheezing, rhonchi, decreased breath sounds
      4. "Staccato cough" in infants with *Chlamydia trachomatis*

III. Pediatric Pneumonia: Diagnosis
   A. Typically a clinical diagnosis
   B. Laboratory and imaging studies helpful to establish etiology or when the case is unclear
      1. Blood and sputum cultures and gram stains if hospitalized
      2. Rapid viral testing
      3. *Mycoplasma* studies
   C. Chest X-ray
      1. Lobar consolidation more likely bacterial
      2. Diffuse interstitial pattern more likely viral
   D. Always include foreign body aspiration in the differential, especially with an acute onset of symptoms and when auscultation is asymmetric

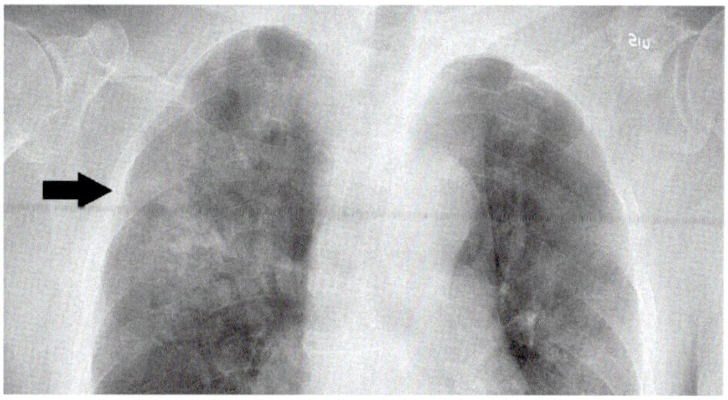

Mikael Häggström, M.D. - Author info - Reusing imagesWritten informed consent was obtained from the individual, including online publication., CC0, via Wikimedia Commons

FIGURE 18.1.101 - Chest X-ray: Patchy Consolidation in Bacterial Pneumonia

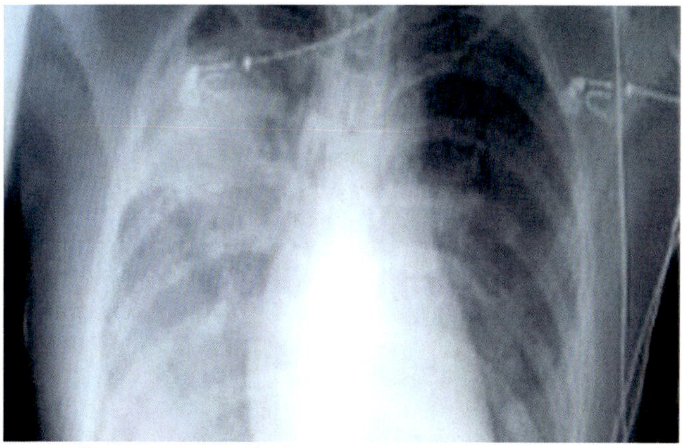

CDC (https://commons.wikimedia.org/wiki/File:SARS_xray.jpg#filelinks), „SARS xray", marked as public domain, more details on Wikimedia Commons: https://commons.wikimedia.org/wiki/Template:PD-US

FIGURE 18.1.102 - Chest X-ray: Bilateral, Diffuse Opacities in Viral Pneumonia

IV. Pediatric Pneumonia: Management
   A. Many can be treated outpatient with supportive care and antimicrobials
      1. Options include amoxicillin, amoxicillin/clavulanate, cephalosporins, macrolides
      2. If influenza, can start neuraminidase inhibitors if < 48 hours since symptom onset
      3. Neuraminidase inhibitors: oseltamivir and zanamivir
   B. Indications for hospitalization
      1. Significant tachypnea or hypoxia
      2. Toxic appearance
      3. Inability to maintain hydration
      4. Complicated pneumonia (abscess, parapneumonic effusion, etc.)
   C. Inpatient management
      1. Supportive care: IV fluids, proper nutrition, antipyretics, supplemental oxygen
      2. If suspecting *Streptococcus pneumoniae,* empiric antibiotics include ampicillin or 3rd generation cephalosporin
      3. If suspecting *Staphylococcus aureus,* empiric antibiotics include clindamycin or vancomycin

D. Treatment typically lasts 7 - 10 days

E. Prevention
1. *Streptococcus pneumoniae* vaccine
2. *Haemophilus influenzae* type B vaccine
3. Influenza vaccination

Condition	Etiology	Key Features
Epiglottitis	- Inflammation of epiglottis and surrounding supraglottis - Most commonly bacterial infection	- Drooling, dysphagia, muffled voice - Tripod position - "Thumbprint" sign on lateral neck X-ray
Croup	- Inflammation of larynx and subglottic airway - Most commonly due to parainfluenza virus	- "Seal-bark" cough - Inspiratory stridor - "Steeple sign" on chest X-ray
Tracheitis	- Invasive exudative bacterial infection of the soft tissues of the trachea - Most commonly associated with *S. aureus, S. pneumoniae*	- Similar findings to croup but does not respond to racemic epinephrine
Pertussis	- Respiratory tract infection due to *Bordetella pertussis* bacteria	- Whooping cough - Lymphocytosis on labs - Catarrhal, paroxysmal, and convalescent stages
Bronchiolitis	- Lower airway viral infection - Most commonly due to RSV	- More severe in premature infants - Primary prevention includes palivizumab in high-risk patients
Pediatric pneumonia	- Inflammatory condition of lungs involving the lung parenchyma - Associated with both viral and bacterial pathogens	- Bacterial pathogens typically cause lobar pneumonia - Viral pathogens typically cause a diffuse, interstitial pneumonia

TABLE 18.1.19 - Infections of the Respiratory Tract

REVIEW QUESTIONS

1. An 11-year-old boy is brought to his primary care physician by his mother due to cough and fever for the last 4 days. Several of his classmates were ill with the same symptoms one week ago. Vital signs include a temperature of 100.5° F (38.1° C), blood pressure of 120/80 mmHg, heart rate of 91 beats/min, and respiratory rate of 15 breaths/min. A rapid influenza test is positive, later confirmed with polymerase chain reaction (PCR). Other notable labs include a mildly elevated ESR. A chest X-ray shows bilateral interstitial opacities. The medical student involved in this patient's care suggests initiation of oseltamivir, but the resident and attending choose not to administer this medication. The patient is also improving clinically. Which of the following is the most likely reason for not initiating this targeted therapy in this particular patient?

    A. A 4-day history of symptoms
    B. Stable vital signs
    C. Low-grade fever
    D. Mild elevation of ESR

- **The correct answer is option A.**
- This patient presents with a low-grade fever and cough.
- His rapid influenza and polymerase chain reaction (PCR) tests returned positive.
- The chest X-ray shows bilateral interstitial opacities.
- All of these findings are consistent with influenza pneumonia.
- Although oseltamivir, a neuraminidase inhibitor, can shorten the duration of illness, its efficacy is well-documented only if given within the first 48 hours of symptom onset.
- However, if the patient had a severe, refractory disease or was immunocompromised, neuraminidase inhibitors would be considered even 48 hours after the onset of symptoms.
- Options B, C, and D are incorrect because none of these factors affect the decision of not initiating oseltamivir as much as the duration of symptoms.

Pediatrics | Section 26: Neonatal Sepsis and Meningitis

I. Neonatal Sepsis: General Characteristics
   A. Clinical syndrome in an infant less than 28 days old with systemic signs of infection and isolation of a bacterial pathogen from the bloodstream
   B. Early-onset
      1. Due to contaminated amniotic fluid or mother's lower genital tract
   C. Late-onset
      1. Vertical transmission or horizontal transmission
   D. Most common pathogens: Group B *Streptococcus, Escherichia coli*
   E. Other potential pathogens include *Listeria monocytogenes, Staphylococcus aureus, Enterococcus,* and *Pseudomonas aeruginosa*
   F. Incidence of early-onset GBS sepsis is declining due to intrapartum prophylaxis
   G. Risk factors
      1. Chorioamnionitis
      2. Intrapartum maternal fever
      3. Preterm delivery (< 37 weeks)
      4. Maternal GBS colonization
      5. Prolonged membrane rupture

II. Neonatal Sepsis: Clinical Features
   A. Nonspecific signs and symptoms
      1. Temperature instability
      2. Irritability, lethargy
      3. Tachypnea, grunting, hypoxia
      4. Poor feeding
      5. Tachycardia
      6. Poor perfusion and hypotension

III. Neonatal Sepsis: Evaluation
   A. Early-onset
      1. History of pregnancy and birth
      2. CBC and blood cultures
      3. Lumbar puncture
      4. Chest X-ray
   B. Late-onset
      1. CBC and blood cultures
      2. Lumbar puncture
      3. Chest X-ray
      4. Urine culture
      5. Cultures from any other potential infection sources

IV. Neonatal Sepsis: Management
   A. Supportive care
      1. Respiratory support
      2. Metabolic support
      3. Fluid and electrolyte support
   B. Empiric antibiotics
      1. Early-onset: ampicillin plus gentamicin (covers GBS, *Listeria, E. Coli)*
      2. Avoid ceftriaxone due to risk of hyperbilirubinemia
      3. Late-onset, community-acquired: ampicillin and gentamicin
      4. Late-onset, hospitalized since birth: vancomycin
      5. Can be narrowed once blood cultures return

V. Neonatal Bacterial Meningitis: General Characteristics
   A. Most common in the first month of life
   B. Most commonly due to group B *Streptococcus, E. coli,* and other gram-negative bacilli
   C. Risk factors
      1. Low birth weight or preterm birth
      2. Premature or prolonged rupture of membranes
      3. Maternal peripartum infection

VI. Neonatal Bacterial Meningitis: Clinical Features
   A. Very similar to neonatal sepsis
      1. Temperature instability
      2. Irritability, lethargy, poor tone, poor feeding
      3. Neurologic symptoms such as tremors, twitching, seizures
      4. Respiratory distress or apnea
      5. Bulging fontanelle and nuchal rigidity not common at initial presentation

VII. Neonatal Bacterial Meningitis: Evaluation
   A. Pregnancy and birth history
   B. Similar work up to sepsis since findings are nonspecific
      1. CBC and blood cultures
      2. Urine cultures
      3. Lumbar puncture with CSF cell count, protein, glucose, gram stain, and culture
      4. Perform before starting antibiotics
   C. LP results in bacterial meningitis
      1. Elevated cell count
      2. Elevated protein
      3. Decreased glucose

VIII. Neonatal Bacterial Meningitis: Management
   A. Supportive care
      1. Respiratory support
      2. IV fluid replacement and nutritional support
      3. Prevent hypoglycemia
      4. Seizure control
   B. Empiric antibiotics
      1. Early-onset and community-acquired late-onset: ampicillin, gentamicin, and a third-generation cephalosporin
      2. Late-onset, hospitalized since birth: vancomycin, aminoglycosides, and extended-generation cephalosporins
      3. Can narrow therapy once cultures isolate a bacterial pathogen

REVIEW QUESTIONS

1. A five-day-old baby boy is brought to the emergency department by his parents because of a fever of 102.7° F (39.2° C) and lethargy for the past day. His parents also note he hasn't been feeding much over the past day. On further examination, his blood pressure is found to be 80/50 mmHg and his heart rate is 155 beats/minute. What is the most likely diagnosis and source of infection?
   - **The most likely diagnosis is neonatal sepsis; the infection source is likely contaminated amniotic fluid or bacteria within the mother's genital tract.**
   - This neonate presents with a high fever, poor feeding, lethargy, hypotension, and tachycardia. These are all features of neonatal sepsis.
   - Since this neonate is less than seven days old, this is early-onset neonatal sepsis and is most likely due to contaminated amniotic fluid or bacteria within the mother's lower genital tract during delivery.

2. If a three-day-old neonate has a positive blood culture and is diagnosed with sepsis, what antibiotic(s) should be started empirically? What pathogens are important to cover with the empirical treatment?
   - **Empiric therapy for early-onset neonatal sepsis is ampicillin plus gentamicin, and the organisms covered are group B *streptococcus, Listeria,* and *E. coli*.**
   - If a neonate less than seven days old is diagnosed with sepsis, it is considered early-onset neonatal sepsis.

3. A 4-month-old infant who has been in the NICU since birth develops a fever of 102.6° F (39.2° C). She has also become more lethargic, irritable, and not feeling well. A lumbar puncture with CSF analysis shows an elevated cell count, elevated protein, and decreased glucose. What therapy should be initiated empirically for this patient?
   - **This patient should be treated empirically with vancomycin, aminoglycosides, and extended-generation cephalosporins.**
   - This infant presents with signs of sepsis.
   - Lumbar puncture shows an elevated cell count, elevated protein, and decreased glucose in the CSF, which is indicative of bacterial meningitis.
   - Since this patient is older than seven days, it is considered late-onset bacterial meningitis and should be treated empirically with vancomycin, aminoglycosides, and extended-generation cephalosporins.

Pediatrics | Section 27: Viral Exanthems

I. Erythema Infectiosum
   A. Due to parvovirus B19
   B. Also known as fifth disease
   C. Mild febrile illness with flu-like symptoms
   D. Two to five days after fever, develop initial diffuse redness of the face with perioral sparing
   E. "Slapped-cheek" rash
   F. Rash spreads to extremities and trunk; confluent and maculopapular
   G. Complications
      1. Can be associated with arthralgias
      2. In children with hemolytic anemias, virus can cause aplastic crisis due to infection of stem cells
      3. In pregnant women, parvovirus B19 can lead to hydrops fetalis in the fetus

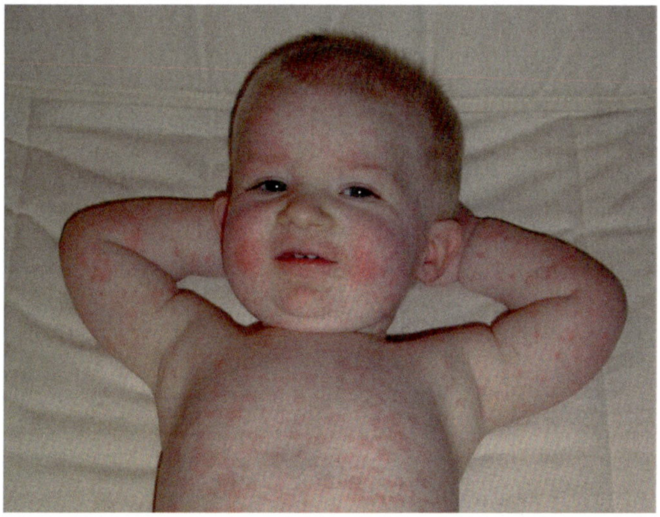

Andrew Kerr, Public domain, via Wikimedia Commons

FIGURE 18.1.103 - Slapped-Cheek Rash of Erythema Infectiosum

I. Measles
   A. Also known as rubeola
   B. Catarrhal stage ("4 C's" of Measles)
      1. Cough
      2. Coryza
      3. Conjunctivitis
      4. Koplik spots
   C. Exanthem stage
      1. One to two days after Koplik spots
      2. Erythematous maculopapular partially confluent rash that begins on the head and spreads downward to the body (cephalocaudal pattern)
      3. Generalized lymphadenopathy
   D. In patients with severe disease, vitamin A supplementation may be used
   E. Subacute sclerosing panencephalitis
      1. Lethal demyelinating inflammation of the brain due to measles infection
      2. Occurs years after initial infection
   F. Included as part of the MMR (measles, mumps, rubella) vaccine

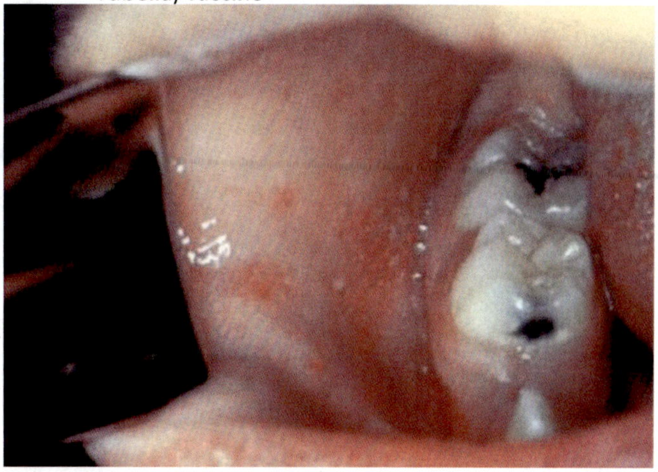

CDC, Public domain, via Wikimedia Commons

FIGURE 18.1.104 - Koplik Spots

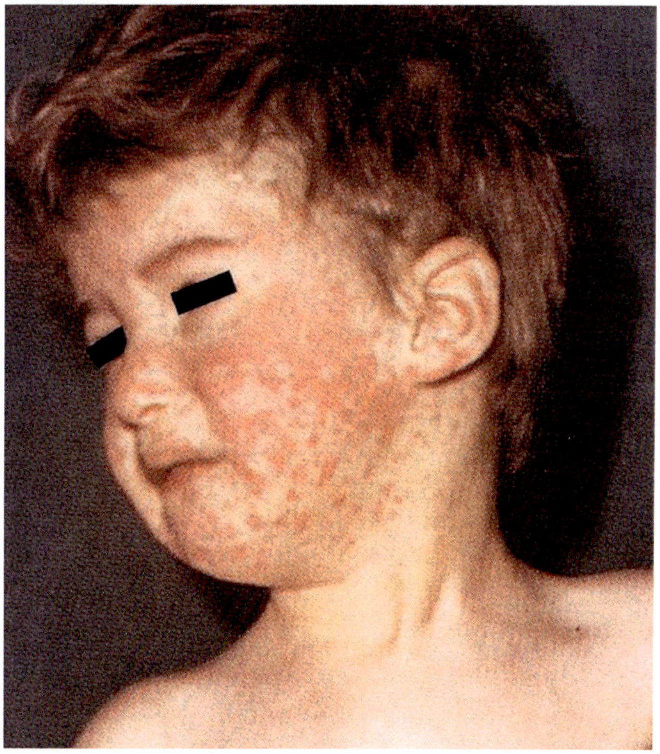

CDC, Public domain, via Wikimedia Commons

FIGURE 18.1.105 - Measles Exanthem

II. Rubella
   A. Also known as German measles
   B. Begins with flu-like symptoms and post-auricular lymphadenopathy
   C. Exanthem phase follows
      1. Fine, nonconfluent maculopapular rash
      2. Starts behind ears and progresses in cephalocaudal pattern
      3. Spares the palms and soles
   D. May also be associated with polyarthritis
   E. Included as part of the MMR vaccine (measles, mumps, rubella)

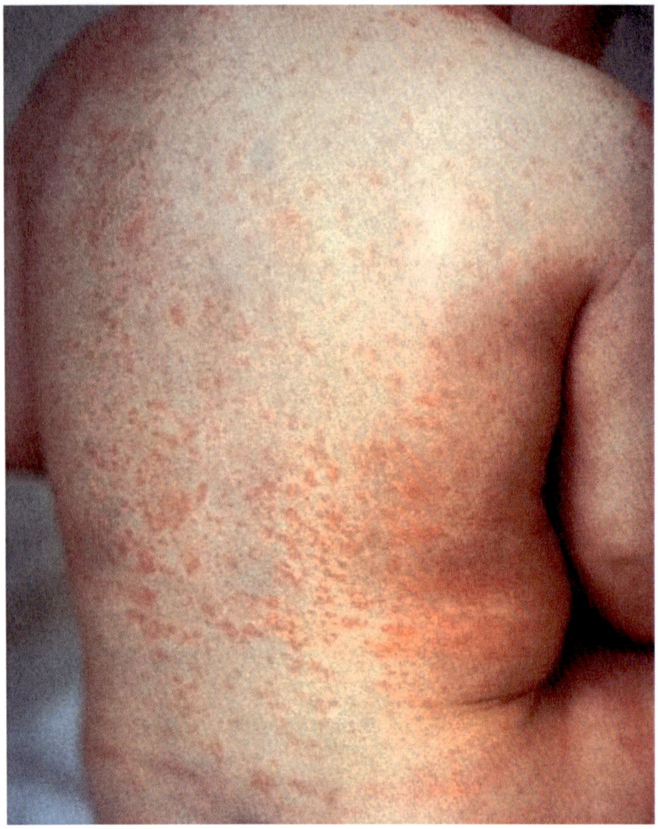

CDC, Public domain, via Wikimedia Commons

FIGURE 18.1.106 - Rubella Exanthem

III. Roseola
   A. Due to human herpesvirus 6 (HHV-6)
   B. Also known as exanthem subitum, sixth disease, three-day fever
   C. Febrile phase
      1. Abrupt onset of high fever, sometimes greater than 104° F
      2. Can result in febrile seizures
      3. Use acetaminophen to reduce fevers
      4. Lasts approximately three days before onset of rash
   D. Exanthem phase
      1. Sudden resolution of temperature
      2. Patchy, maculopapular rash
      3. Sometimes described as rose-colored or lacy in appearance
      4. Originates on trunk and spreads to extremities

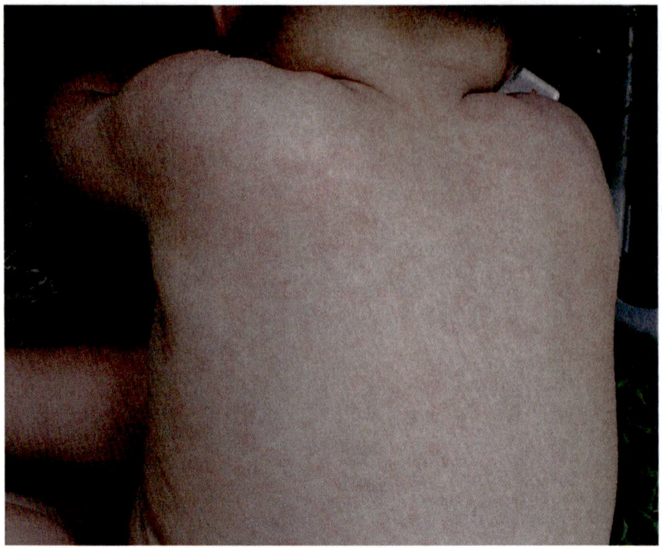

Emiliano Burzagli, Public domain, via Wikimedia Commons

FIGURE 18.1.107 - Roseola Exanthem

IV. Varicella
   A. Also known as chickenpox
   B. Highly contagious
   C. Prodromal phase one to two days before the exanthem
      1. Fever, malaise
      2. Some children may not have this phase
   D. Exanthem phase
      1. Starts on the trunk and spreads to face and extremities
      2. Severely pruritic
      3. Begins as erythematous macules, progresses to vesicles filled with clear fluid that rupture and crust over
      4. Hallmark of the exanthem is multiple stages of the rash present at once
   E. Most patients just need supportive care with calamine lotion or oral antihistamines
   F. In immunocompromised patients, acyclovir may be required
   G. Vaccine is available to prevent disease

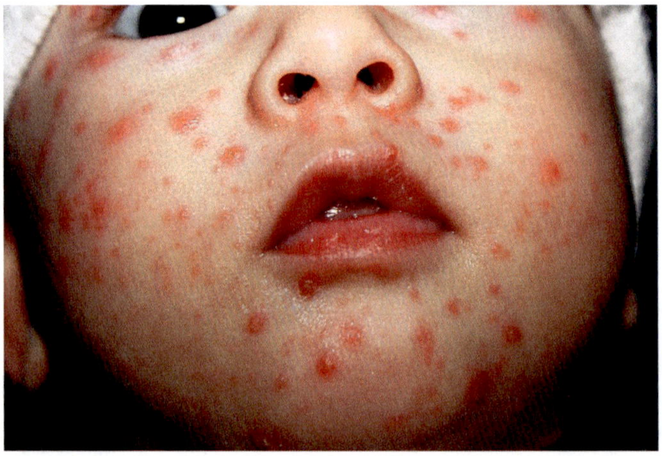

Øyvind Holmstad, CC BY-SA 4.0 <https://creativecommons.org/licenses/by-sa/4.0>, via Wikimedia Commons

FIGURE 18.1.108 - Varicella Exanthem

Condition	Key Features
Erythema infectiosum	- Parvovirus B19 - "Slapped-cheek" rash - Aplastic anemia in patients with hemolytic anemias - Hydrops fetalis in pregnant mothers
Measles	- Cough, coryza, conjunctivitis, Koplik spots - Erythematous maculopapular rash that spreads in cephalocaudal pattern - Subacute sclerosing panencephalitis years later
Rubella	- Postauricular lymphadenopathy and flu-like symptoms - Fine nonconfluent maculopapular rash - Spreads in cephalocaudal pattern
Roseola	- Human herpesvirus 6 - Begins with very high fevers - May be associated with febrile seizures - Fever resolves and lacy pink rash appears
Varicella	- Highly pruritic - Rash in different stages of healing - Macules, fluid-filled vesicles, crusted papules

TABLE 18.1.20 - Viral Exanthems

REVIEW QUESTIONS

1. A 4-year-old girl is brought to the emergency department by her mother because of cough, rhinorrhea, and conjunctivitis. The family recently immigrated from Vietnam and she is not up to date on all of her vaccinations. Physical examination shows white spots on the buccal mucosa. What is the most likely diagnosis?
    - **The most likely diagnosis is rubeola.**
    - This 4-year-old girl recently immigrated and is not up to date on her vaccinations.
    - She has a cough, rhinorrhea, and conjunctivitis with physical examination notable for spots on the buccal mucosa concerning for measles.
    - The white spots on the buccal mucosa are called Koplik spots.
    - Therefore, this girl likely has measles, also known as rubeola, which will be treated symptomatically.

2. An 18-month-old boy is brought to the clinic by his mother because of generalized body aches and flu-like symptoms that began several days ago. Physical examination shows a fever of 102.1° F (38.9° C) and a maculopapular rash. His mother states that the rash began on the head and spread downward, sparing the palms and soles. Additionally, lymphadenopathy is present behind the child's ears bilaterally. Upon additional history, the family notes they recently immigrated from Mexico, and the child is not up to date on all of his vaccinations. What is the most likely diagnosis?

    A. Rubeola
    B. Varicella
    C. Roseola
    D. Rubella

    - **The correct answer is option D.**
    - This 18-month-old boy presents with flu-like symptoms and a maculopapular rash that started on his head.
    - He is not up to date on all of his vaccinations.
    - Physical examination also revieals postauricular lymphadenopathy, consistent with rubella, also called German measles.
    - Option A is incorrect because rubeola presents with a similar rash but patients tend to have the 4 C's: cough, coryza, conjunctivitis, and Koplik spots.
    - Option B is incorrect because varicella aka chicken pox presents with a rash starting on the trunk and spreading outward. Varicella also shows a rash in mixed stages of macules, then vesicles, which then rupture and crust over.
    - Option C is incorrect because roseola typically presents as an abrupt high fever, which lasts 3 days and resolves as a rose-colored lacy rash.

Pediatrics | Section 28: Well-Child Care

I. Introduction
  A. Bright Futures recommends that each well-child visit consists of:
    1. Observation (e.g. child behavior, parent-child interaction)
    2. Physical examination
    3. Screening
    4. Immunizations
    5. Anticipatory guidance

II. Anticipatory Guidance
  A. Clinicians provide guidance to caregivers
    1. Child safety, relationship issues, access to community services
    2. Age-specific
  B. Commonly-tested points
    1. Have the baby sleep supine to reduce the risk of SIDS
    2. Avoid placing objects in the crib with the baby (e.g. toys)
    3. Use rear-facing car seat until age 2 years and weighs 40 pounds
    4. Introduce solid foods beginning at 6 months old
    5. Don't introduce cow's milk until 12 months old to prevent anemia
    6. Set the water heater temperature < 48.8° C (120° F)
    7. Lock medications and household cleaning products up
    8. Do not administer ipecac after an accidental poison ingestion
      a) Increases risk of further damage to the esophagus
    9. Cover power outlets, use safety gates on stairs
    10. Fire: ensure smoke detectors in the home are functional
    11. Water: observe children around water at all times, use life jackets, teach children to swim, and fence around any pools
    12. Guns: if present in home, store locked and unloaded

III. Hearing Screening
  a. All newborns should be screened
  A. Trouble with articulation and language skills may be a sign of underlying hearing loss
  B. Most common cause of non-hereditary hearing loss in children is congenital cytomegalovirus infection
    1. May cause unilateral or bilateral hearing impairment
  C. Chronic otitis media and middle ear effusions can cause hearing loss

Condition	Etiologies	Screening Recommendations
Hearing	- Congenital (e.g. cytomegalovirus) - Acquired (e.g. otitis media)	- Screen all newborns before hospital discharge - Otoacoustic emission or auditory brainstem response
Iron-deficiency anemia	- Cow's milk impairs iron absorption and contains little iron	- Hemoglobin in every child at 12 months old
Lead poisoning	- Lead paint, contaminated drinking water, ammunition	- Blood lead levels - Screen children who are at a high risk of exposure
Hyperlipidemia	- Familial hyperlipidemia - Secondary hyperlipidemia (e.g. nephrotic syndrome)	- Once at 9 - 11 years old - Again at 17 - 21 years old
Drug and alcohol use		- Annual CRAFFT questionnaire - Begin at 11 years old
Depression		- Annual PHQ-2 - Begin at 12 years old

TABLE 18.1.21 - Common Screening Recommendations

Vaccine	Administration	Key Points
Hepatitis B	- First dose hours after birth - Second dose at 2 months - Third dose at 6 months	- Add Hepatitis B immune globulin if the mother is positive for Hepatitis B or if status is unknown
Diphtheria and tetanus toxoids, acellular pertussis (DTaP)	- 2, 4, and 6 months - Fourth dose at 15 - 18 months - Fifth dose at 4 - 6 years	
Inactivated polio	- 2, 4, and 6 months	
Rotavirus	- 2, 4, and 6 months	- Contraindicated in patients with a history of intussusception
Haemophilus influenzae type b (Hib)	- 2, 4, and 6 months - Fourth dose at 12 - 15 months	
Pneumococcal conjugate vaccine (PCV13)	- 2, 4, and 6 months - Fourth dose at 12 - 15 months	- One dose in high-risk patients who are 7 years old or older if not previously vaccinated (e.g. sickle cell disease, splenectomy)
Meningococcal conjugate	- First dose at 11 - 12 years - Booster dose at 16 - 18 years	
Hepatitis A	- Two doses at least 6 months apart - Administer between ages 12 - 24 months old	
Inactivated influenza	- Annually beginning at 6 months old	
Measles, mumps, rubella (MMR)	- First dose at 12 - 15 months - Second dose at 4 - 6 years	- Febrile seizures - Vaccine strain measles virus → fever and maculopapular rash
Varicella	- First dose at 12 - 15 months - Second dose at 4 - 6 years	- Vaccine strain varicella → maculopapular or vesicular rash that can be contagious

TABLE 18.1.22 - Key Immunizations

Birth	2 mo.	4 mo.	6 mo.	1 yr.	15 mo.	18 mo.	4 yr.	11 yr.	16 yr.
Hep. B	Hep. B		Hep. B						
	DTaP	DTaP	DTaP		DTaP		DTaP		
	Polio	Polio	Polio						
	Rotavirus	Rotavirus	Rotavirus						
	HiB	HiB	HiB	HiB					
	PCV13	PCV13	PCV13	PCV13					
				Hep. A		Hep. A			
			Influenza (yearly)						
				MMR			MMR		
				Varicella			Varicella		
								Meningococcal conjugate	Meningococcal conjugate

TABLE 18.1.23 - Immunization Schedule

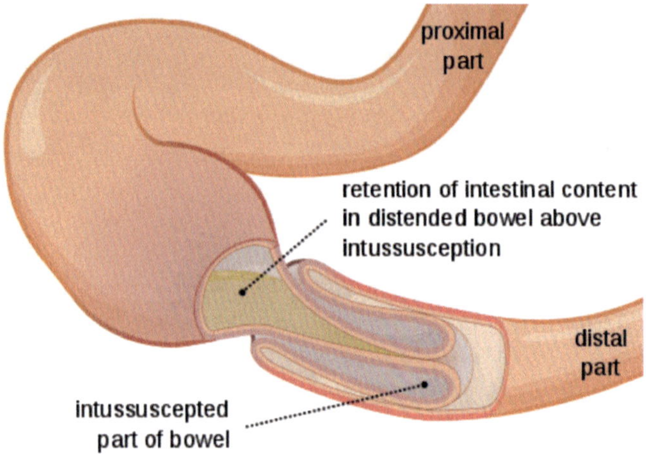

FIGURE 18.1.109 - Intussusception

IV. Immunizations
   A. Live-attenuated vaccines
      1. Rotavirus
      2. Measles, mumps, rubella (MMR)
      3. Varicella
      4. Intranasal influenza vaccine
      5. Yellow fever
   B. Contraindications to immunizations
      1. Live-attenuated vaccines are contraindicated in children under 1 year old, immunosuppression, and pregnancy
      2. Rotavirus vaccine if there is a history of intussusception
      3. Pertussis vaccine if previous dose caused encephalopathy
      4. Hepatitis B if the newborn weighs < 2 kg (< 4.4 lbs)
      5. Any true allergy to a component of the vaccine
   C. Not contraindications
      1. A low-grade fever or mild illness
      2. Current antibiotic use
      3. Prematurity (e.g. administer based on chronological age)
   D. Egg allergy
      1. Administer MMR and influenza vaccines with observation
      2. Administer the yellow fever vaccine with caution

REVIEW QUESTIONS

1. Which immunizations should be given to otherwise healthy children at 2 months?
   - **At 2 months, children should receive a second dose of hepatitis B, DTaP, inactivated polio, rotavirus, Haemophilus influenzae type b, and pneumococcal conjugate vaccine or PCV13.**

2. A 1-year-old boy is brought to his primary care physician by his mother for a well-child exam. He was born at 34 weeks gestation via spontaneous vaginal delivery. He was diagnosed with acute otitis media 2 days ago, and he has been taking oral amoxicillin since then. Vital signs include temperature of 100.4° F (38° C), blood pressure of 89/70 mmHg, heart rate of 95 mmHg, and respiratory rate of 17 breaths/min. Physical examination is unremarkable. The physician suggests he receive his first dose of the MMR vaccine. The mother is hesitant about vaccines due to her personal beliefs. The physician discusses the risks and benefits of vaccination as well as its contraindications. If the physician obtains parental consent, which of the following is the best next step in the management of this patient?

   A. Administer vaccine now
   B. Administer vaccine once afebrile
   C. Administer vaccine once antibiotics are discontinued
   D. Administer vaccine after 6 weeks

   - **The correct answer is option A.**
   - This 1-year-old boy presents on a well-child visit.
   - He was born prematurely at 34 weeks gestation via spontaneous vaginal delivery.
   - He was diagnosed with acute otitis media 2 days ago, and he has been taking oral amoxicillin.
   - Vital signs are significant for a low-grade fever of 38° C (100.4° F).
   - The physician suggests the patient receive his first dose of the MMR vaccine. However, the mother is hesitant about vaccines due to her personal beliefs.
   - If the physician obtains parental consent after this conversation, he should administer the vaccine now. This is because prematurity, low-grade fever, and current antibiotic use are not contraindications for vaccine administration.
   - Options B and C are incorrect because fever and current antibiotic use are not contraindications for vaccine administration.
   - Option D is incorrect because although this patient was born at 34 weeks of gestation, he should receive vaccinations based on his chronological age rather than the corrected gestational age.

Pediatrics | Section 29: Well-Child Care - Physical Exam

Measurement	Key Components	Common Pathologies
Blood pressure	- Normal range differs with age	- Hypotension (e.g. dehydration, sepsis) - Hypertension (e.g. renal disease, endocrine disease)
Temperature	- Normal temperature is 35 - 38° C (95 - 100.3° F)	- Sepsis → hyperthermia or hypothermia - A fever in an infant is a medical emergency
Heart rate	- Normal range differs with age - > 100 beats/min is not uncommon	- Tachycardia (e.g. dehydration, infection) - Bradycardia (e.g. hypothermia, structural heart disease)
Respiratory rate	- Normal differs with age - > 20 breaths/min is not uncommon	- Tachypnea (e.g. pneumonia, transient tachypnea of the newborn) - Apnea (e.g. apnea of prematurity, brief resolved unexplained event [BRUE])
Growth measurements	- Height, weight, and head circumference - Crossing 2 or more percentile lines is a red flag	- Growth delay (e.g. malnutrition) - Growth acceleration (e.g. hydrocephalus, precocious puberty)

TABLE 18.1.24 - Vital Signs and Growth Measurements

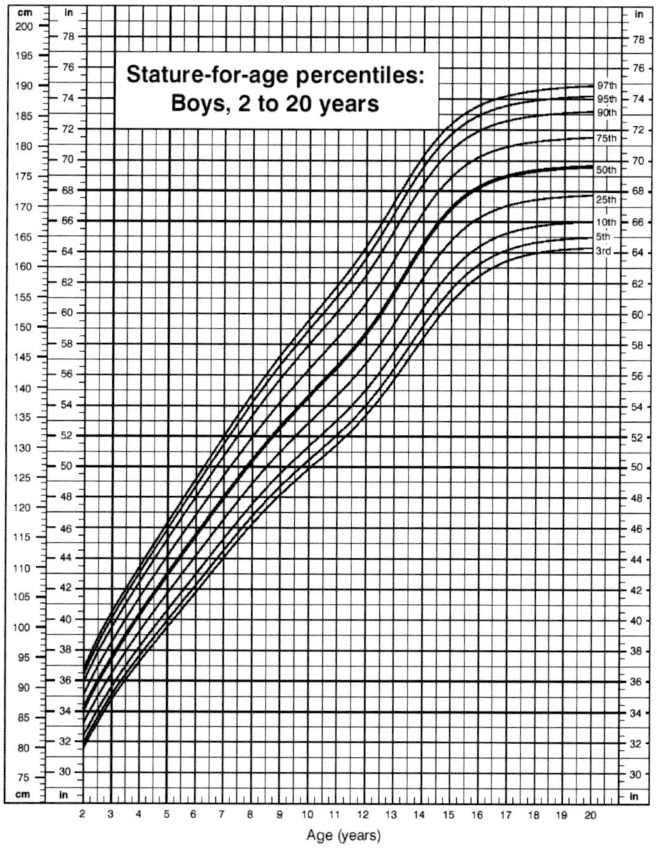

CDC/Public Domain

FIGURE 18.1.110 - Pediatric Growth Chart

Examination portion	Key Components	Common Pathologies
Head	- Assess for cranial birth injuries - Fontanelles	- Caput succedaneum, cephalohematoma, subgaleal hemorrhage
Eyes	- Alignment - Red reflex	- Strabismus, amblyopia - Retinoblastoma, cataracts
Ears	- The top of the helix should be at the level of the outer canthus of the eye	- Low-set ears (e.g. Down syndrome, Edward syndrome)
Nose	- Assess the shape and patency - Note discharge	- Choanal atresia causes the face to turn blue when feeding - A foreign body causes unilateral purulent discharge
Heart	- Auscultate for murmurs - Differentiate whether the murmur is benign or pathologic	- Benign murmurs (e.g. Still murmur) - Pathologic murmur (e.g. Tetralogy of Fallot)
Lungs	- Assess work of breathing - Auscultate for wheezing or inspiratory stridor	- Wheezing (e.g. asthma) - Inspiratory stridor (e.g. laryngomalacia, croup)
Abdomen	- Note any protrusion or scaphoid appearance - Auscultate bowel sounds, assess organ size, identify areas of tenderness	- Protruded abdomen (e.g. necrotizing enterocolitis) - Scaphoid abdomen (e.g. diaphragmatic hernia) - Enlarged organ size (e.g. malignancy)
Genitourinary	- Assess normal structure of the genitals - Look for rashes in the diaper area	- Cryptorchidism, epi/hypospadias, labial adhesions - Diaper dermatitis, Candida dermatitis
Lower extremities	- Femoral pulses - Barlow and Ortolani maneuvers; Galeazzi sign - Assess normal structure of the feet and ankles	- Weak femoral pulses (e.g. aortic coarctation) - Congenital hip dysplasia - Club foot, metatarsus adductus
Spine	- Sacral dimple - Spine curvature	- Spina bifida - Scoliosis
Neurologic	- Developmental reflexes (e.g. Moro, Palmar, Plantar, Rooting)	- Neurologic dysfunction
Skin	- Head-to-toe skin examination	- Congenital dermal melanocytosis (Mongolian spot) - Acne vulgaris

TABLE 18.1.25 - Key Features of Pediatric Physical Examination

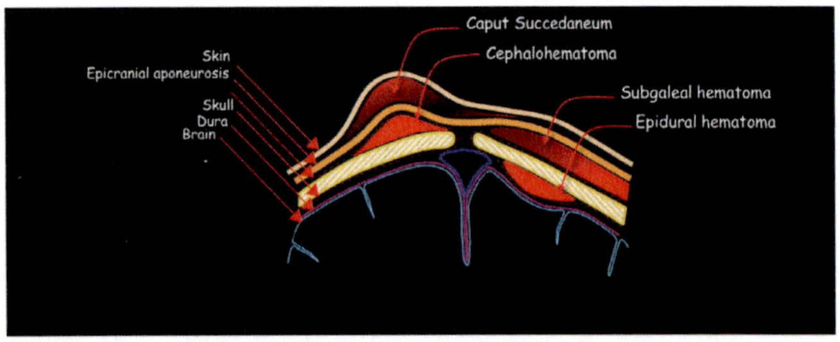

FIGURE 18.1.111- Cranial Birth Injuries

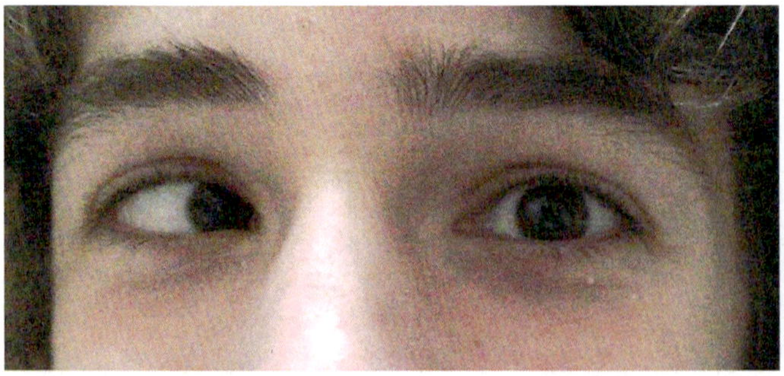

FIGURE 18.1.112 - Strabismus

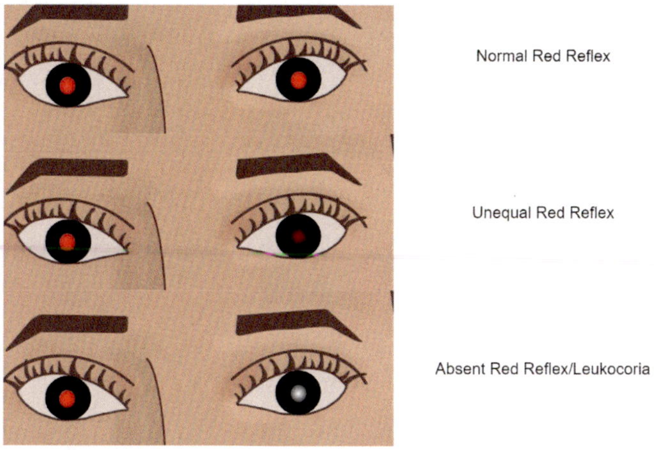

FIGURE 18.1.113 - Normal Red Reflex vs. Abnormal Red Reflex

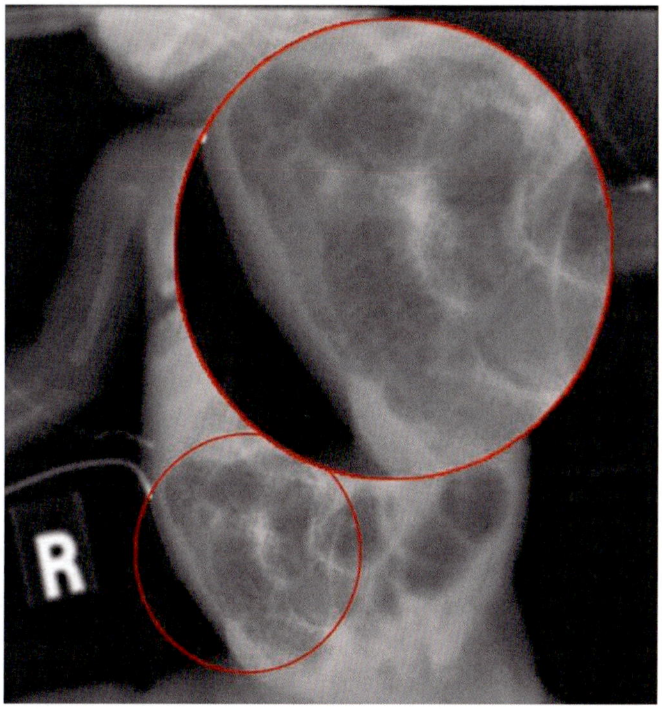

FIGURE 18.1.114 - Abdominal X-ray: Pneumatosis Intestinalis

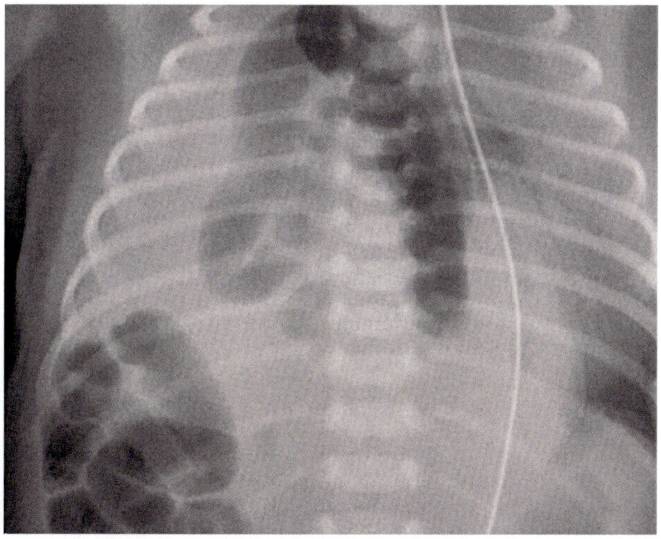

FIGURE 18.1.115 - X-ray: Congenital Diaphragmatic Hernia

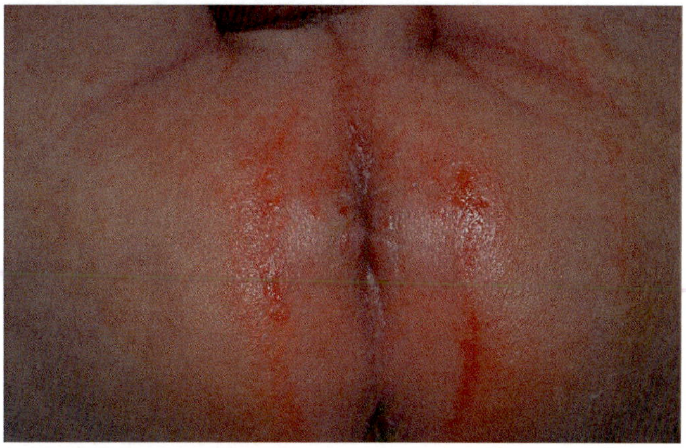

FIGURE 18.1.116 - Irritant Diaper Dermatitis

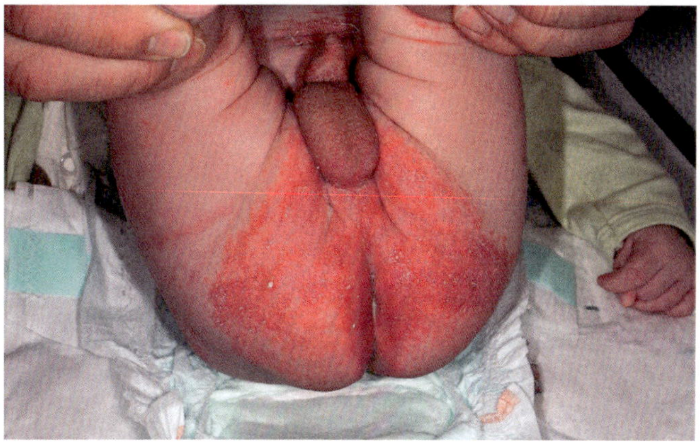

FIGURE 18.1.117 - *Candida* Diaper Dermatitis

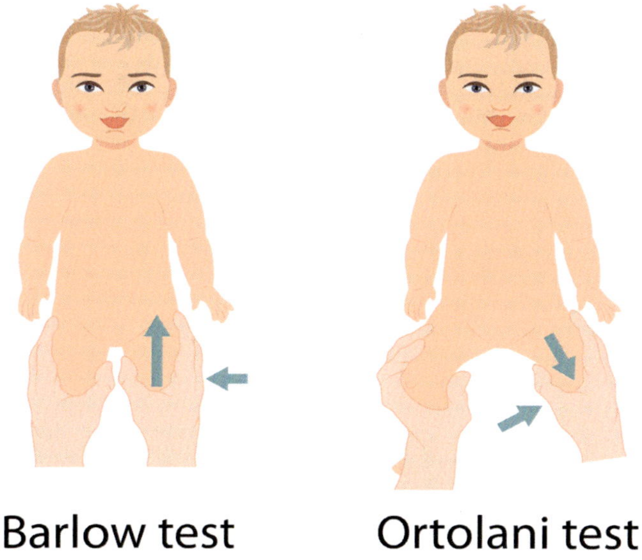

FIGURE 18.1.118 - Barlow & Ortolani Tests

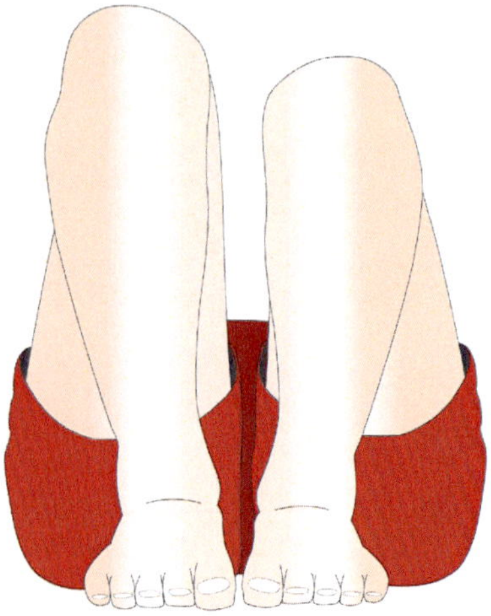

FIGURE 18.1.119 - Galeazzi Sign

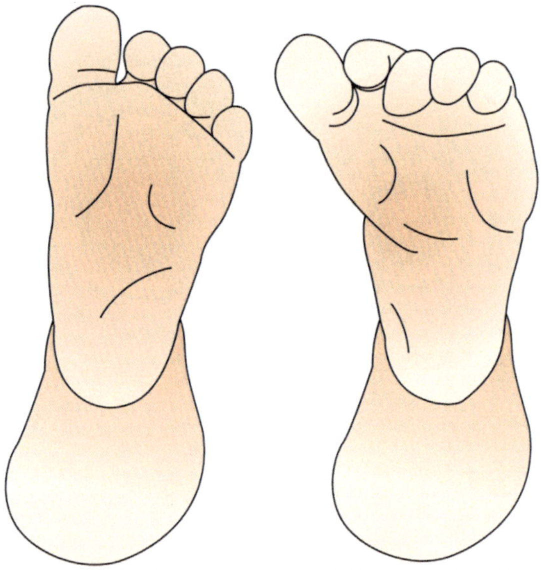

FIGURE 18.1.121 - Metatarsus Adductus

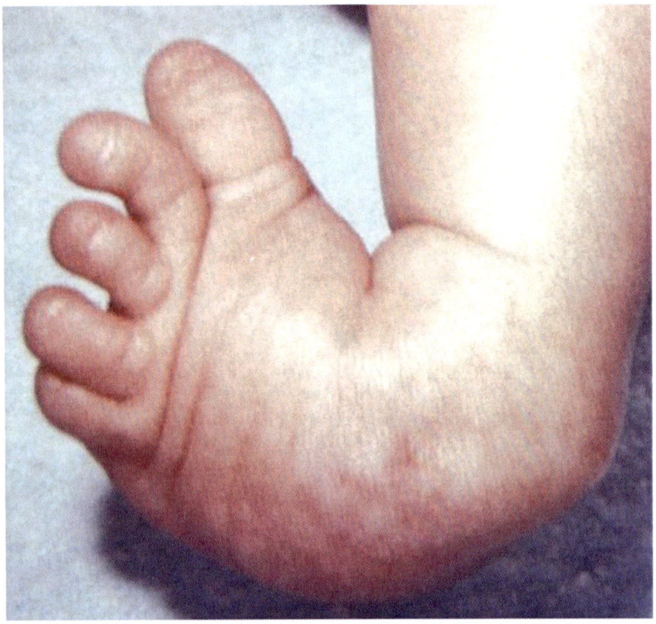

FIGURE 18.1.120 - Club Foot

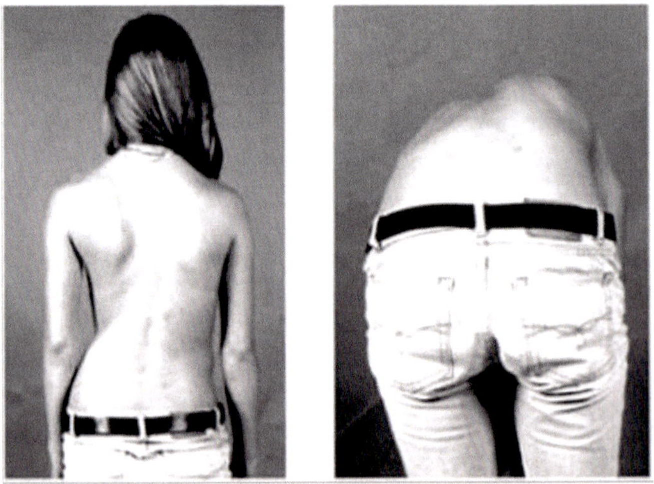

FIGURE 18.1.122 - "Rib-Humping" Sign in Scoliosis

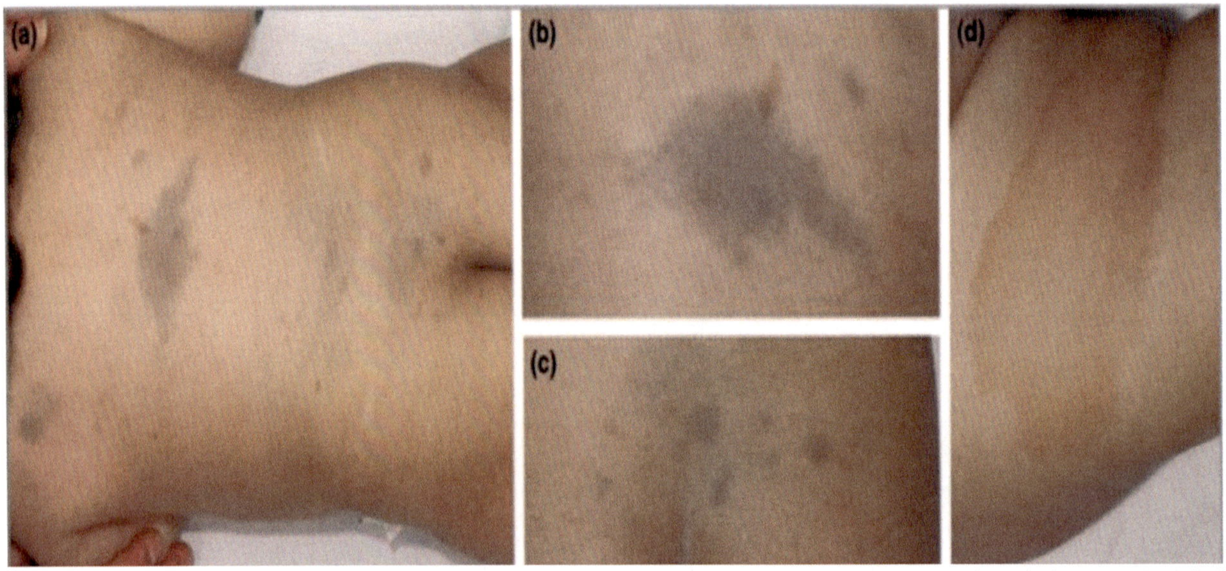

FIGURE 18.1.123 - Congenital Dermal Melanocytosis

REVIEW QUESTIONS

1. A 3-year-old girl is brought to her primary care physician by her mom for a well-child visit. Physical examination shows a medially-deviated left eye and asymmetric pupillary red reflexes. What is the next best step in diagnosis?
    - **The next best step in diagnosis is a fundoscopic examination.**
    - This girl has a medially-deviated left eye, or strabismus, and asymmetric pupillary red reflexes.
    - Both of these findings may be signs of an insidious ocular pathology, such as retinoblastoma, which would become more evident on a careful fundoscopic examination.

2. Physical examination of a 2-month-old girl shows a positive Ortolani test and a positive Galeazzi test. What is the next best step in diagnosis?
    - **The next best step in diagnosis is an ultrasound of both hips.**
    - Physical examination of this 2-month-old girl shows a positive Ortolani test and a positive Galeazzi test, which is suggestive of developmental dysplasia of the hip.
    - If developmental dysplasia of the hip is suspected in a child less than 4 months old, clinicians should strongly consider a follow-up ultrasound of the hip.
    - If, however, the condition is suspected in a child older than 4 months old, clinicians should obtain a hip radiograph instead in order to properly evaluate the joint.

3. A 3-month-old boy is brought to his primary care physician by his parents due to a foot deformity. They thought it would resolve spontaneously but there is no change in foot position. The patient was born at 39 weeks of gestation via spontaneous vaginal delivery. There were no prenatal or perinatal complications. His vital signs are unremarkable. The physical examination shows bilaterally plantar flexed feet with soles facing superomedially. The midfoot and forefoot are fixated in this position. Which of the following is the most likely diagnosis in this patient?

    A. Scoliosis
    B. Developmental hip dysplasia
    C. Clubfoot
    D. Metatarsus adductus

    - **The correct answer is option C.**
    - This 3-month-old boy presents with foot deformity.
    - The physical examination shows bilaterally plantar flexed feet with soles facing superomedially. This is a classic description of clubfoot, also known as talipes equinovarus.
    - Clubfoot is a congenital musculoskeletal disorder resulting from distorted alignment of ankle and foot bones. It is not likely to resolve spontaneously so it should be corrected either with a cast or a surgery.
    - Option A is incorrect because while scoliosis can result in foot deformities like pes planus or pes cavus, it is not associated with severe misalignment of ankle and foot bones.
    - Option B is incorrect because developmental hip dysplasia presents with positive Ortolani and Barlow tests and Galeazzi signs rather than a foot deformity.
    - Option D is incorrect because metatarsus adductus is characterized by medially deviated metatarsal bones. There is no plantar flexion in metatarsus adductus. Additionally, the midfoot and forefoot are movable rather than fixated in one position.

Pediatrics | Section 30: Child Abuse

I. Child Abuse: Definition
   A. Physical, sexual, and/or psychological mistreatment of a child
   B. Neglect of a child's needs
   C. Any act or failure to act by a caregiver that results in actual or potential harm to a child

II. Child Abuse: Parental Risk Factors
   A. History of alcohol use disorder or substance use disorder
   B. Low education level
   C. Young or single parent
   D. History of mental illness
   E. History of child abuse
   F. Difficult home environment: financial difficulty, domestic violence
   G. Non-parent caregiver

III. Child Abuse: Child Risk Factors
   A. Infants with colic (excessive crying > 3 hours/day, > 3 days/week)
   B. Complex medical problems
   C. Unplanned pregnancy
   D. Multiple hospitalizations

IV. Child Abuse: History
   A. Inconsistent with pattern of injury
   B. Inconsistent or vague story
   C. Delayed in obtaining appropriate medical care
   D. New change in behavior
   E. Child preoccupied with or has excessive knowledge of adult sexual behaviors

V. Child Abuse Presentation: Bruises
   A. Most common physical finding
   B. Located on head or torso
   C. May be in pattern reflecting instrument used for injury (e.g. shape of hand or belt)
   D. Mimics: congenital dermal melanocytosis (Mongolian spots), coining, cupping, bleeding disorders

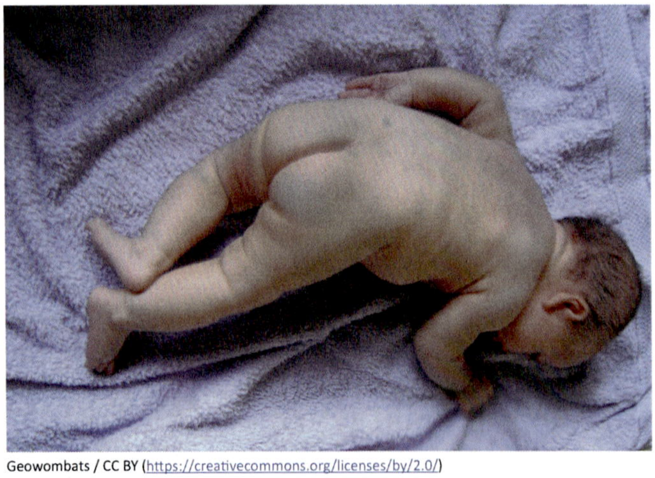

FIGURE 18.1.124 - Congenital Dermal Melanocytosis

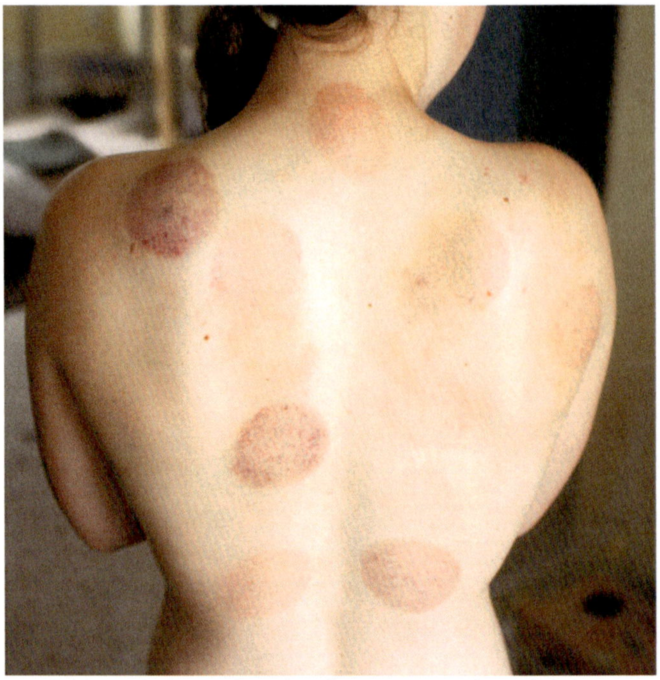

FIGURE 18.1.125 - Cupping Bruises

VI. Child Abuse Presentation: Burns
   A. Well-circumscribed
      1. Contact burns: cigarette, curling iron
      2. Absence of burns in distribution of splash marks
   B. Immersion burns from hot water on buttocks, back, legs
      1. Flexor surfaces spared
   C. Stocking-glove distribution
   D. Mimics: scalded skin syndrome, severe contact dermatitis

VII. Child Abuse Presentation: Fractures
   A. Spiral fractures: rotational or twisting force
      1. Humerus, femur
   B. Epiphyseal or metaphyseal "bucket-handle" fractures
      1. Children < 2 years
   C. Posterior rib fractures
   D. Mimic: osteogenesis imperfecta (blue sclerae, hearing loss, opalescent teeth)

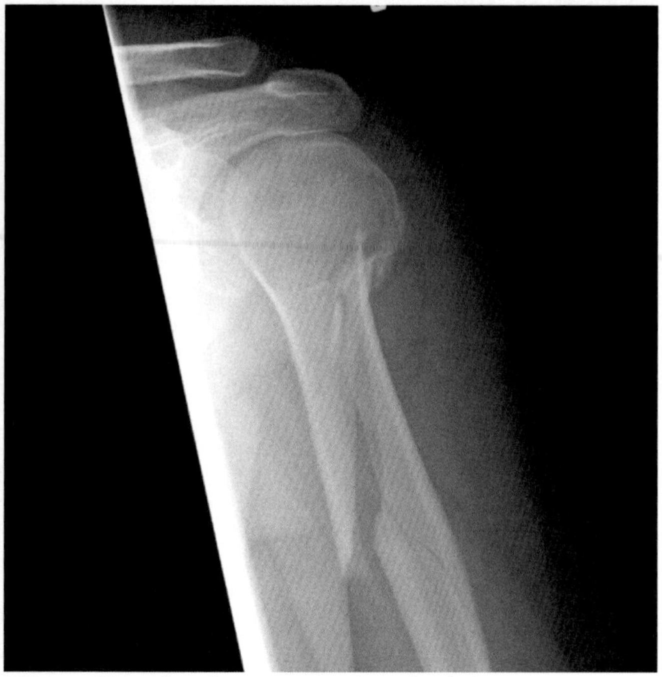

FIGURE 18.1.126 - X-ray of the Humerus: Spiral Fracture

VIII. Child Abuse Presentation: Nonaccidental Head Trauma
- A. Shaken baby syndrome
- B. Brain injury: large head, weak neck muscles, soft brain, low myelination
- C. Lethargy, difficulty feeding, apnea, seizures
- D. Subdural/epidural hematoma → bulging fontanelle
- E. Retinal hemorrhage +/- papilledema
- F. Mimics: accidental head trauma

IX. Child Abuse: Diagnosis
- A. Weight and height
- B. Physical abuse → X-ray skeletal survey
- C. Sexual abuse → STI and sperm testing
- D. Head trauma → noncontrast CT head, ophthalmic exam
  1. MRI for white-matter changes associated with violent shaking

X. Child Abuse: Treatment
- A. Thorough documentation of all injuries
- B. Notify child protective services immediately
  1. Child may need to be removed from home
- C. Hospitalize if necessary
- D. Treat specific injuries
  1. Antibiotics, oral contraceptives, casting, skin/wound care

Age	Normal Sexual Behavior	Abnormal Sexual Behavior
Toddler	Exploring own or other's genitals Masturbatory movements Undressing self or others	Repeated insertion of objects into vagina or anus Sex play involving genital-genital, oral-genital, or anal-genital contact Use of force, threats, or bribes in sex play Age-inappropriate sexual knowledge Preoccupation with sex and masturbation
School-age	Increased interest in sex words and play Asking questions about sex and reproduction Masturbatory movements	

TABLE 18.1.26 - Normal vs. Abnormal Sexual Behaviors of Toddlers and School-Aged Children

REVIEW QUESTIONS

1. A 4-year-old girl is brought to her primary care physician by her mother for a routine examination. Her mother states that she has started preschool and seems to interact well with her peers. She is able to hop on one foot and communicates well with her family, including telling stories. Her mother is concerned that she seems to be talking to imaginary friends and wonders if this is normal. She is also concerned that her daughter is taking too much interest in sex, including touching her and her 2-year-old sister's genitals and asking where babies come from. What is the best course of action with regard to this mother's concerns?

- **The best step in addressing this mother's concerns is to provide reassurance that her daughter's behavior is normal.**
- This healthy 4-year-old girl appears to be meeting her developmental milestones, including hopping on one foot and telling stories.
- Her mother is concerned that she is talking to imaginary friends. However, this is also age-appropriate behavior.
- Her sexual behavior is also age-appropriate, including touching her and her sister's genitals and expressing more interest in sex and reproduction.
- Concerning sexual behavior in children of this age includes insertion of objects into the vagina or anus, sex play involving genital-genital, oral-genital, or anal-genital contact, the use of force, threats, or bribes in sex play, age-inappropriate sexual knowledge, or preoccupation with sex and masturbation. This child has none of these behaviors and, therefore, shows no evidence of abuse.

2. A 2-month-old boy is brought to the emergency department because of lethargy and difficulty feeding for the last 4 hours. His mother states that she left him with her younger brother last night, who reported no issues. However, she noticed a lack of alertness and difficulty feeding this morning. Physical examination shows a sleepy-appearing infant who withdraws to pain but is otherwise minimally responsive. The patient's fontanelle is tense and bulging. What is the next best step in the evaluation of this patient?

   A. X-ray skeletal survey
   B. Ophthalmic exam
   C. Lumbar puncture
   D. Basic metabolic panel
   E. Contact the uncle for a more thorough history

- **The correct answer is option B.**
- The patient has signs and symptoms of traumatic brain injury, including lethargy, difficulty feeding, and a bulging fontanelle after being left with his uncle overnight.
- This is a classic case of abusive head trauma
- The most important next step is to evaluate for non-accidental or abusive head trauma, which is done by performing an ophthalmic exam to look for evidence of retinal hemorrhage and a head CT to assess for subdural or epidural hemorrhage.
- Option A is incorrect because while an X-ray skeletal survey could be helpful in determining other injuries, this patient has signs of head trauma that need to be addressed first.
- Option C is incorrect because the patient has a history suspicious for abusive head trauma rather than infection.
- Option D is incorrect because this patient's symptoms are more likely to have been caused by an abusive head trauma rather than an electrolyte abnormality.
- Option E is incorrect because there's no guarantee that the uncle would be truthful about his care of the infant.

Pediatrics | Section 31: Acute Lymphoblastic Leukemia

I. Acute Lymphoblastic Leukemia: General Features
   A. Malignancy of immature lymphoblasts
   B. Due to block in early development of T cells or B cells
   C. Pre-T cell ALL and pre-B cell ALL (most common)
      1. Pre-T cell ALL: terminal deoxynucleotidyl transferase (TdT) positive
      2. Pre-B cell ALL: TdT and CD10 positive

II. Acute Lymphoblastic Leukemia: Chromosomal Abnormalities
   A. Translocation *12;21* (most common) resulting in *TEL-AML1* fusion gene; better prognosis
   B. *TEL-AML1* inhibits differentiation of lymphoblasts
   C. Translocation *9;22* (Philadelphia chromosome) resulting in *BCR-ABL* fusion gene; worse prognosis
   D. Mutated tyrosine kinase most commonly implicated in CML

III. Acute Lymphoblastic Leukemia: Clinical Presentation
   A. Fatigue and low-grade fever; association with Down syndrome
   B. Increased bleeding tendency
   C. Hepatosplenomegaly and generalized lymphadenopathy
   D. Bone pain (bone metastasis); CNS and testicular metastasis
   E. Mediastinal metastasis in adolescents causing tracheal, esophageal or superior vena cava compression (pre-T ALL)

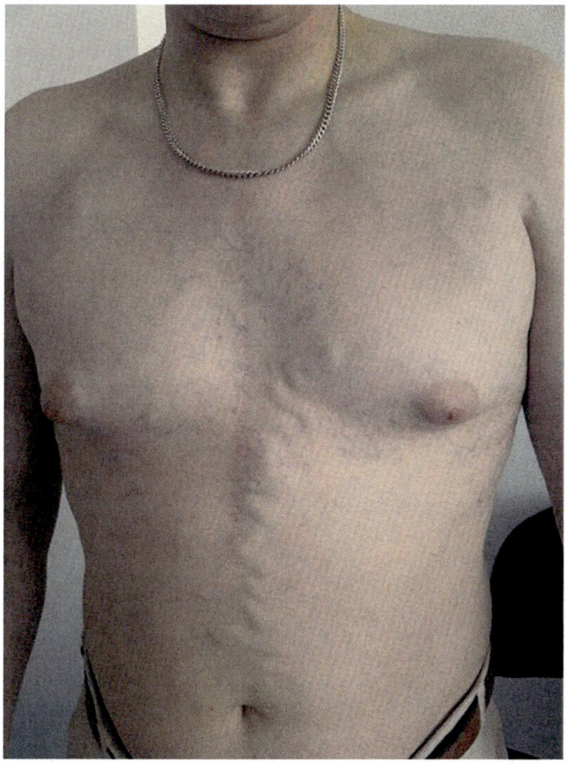

FIGURE 18.1.127 - Patient With Superior Vena Cava Syndrome

IV. Acute Lymphoblastic Leukemia: Diagnosis
   A. Complete blood count with white blood cell differential: absolute lymphocytosis
   B. Peripheral blood smear: lymphoblasts; complete blood count
   C. Bone marrow biopsy: > 20% of lymphoblasts (vs. chronic)

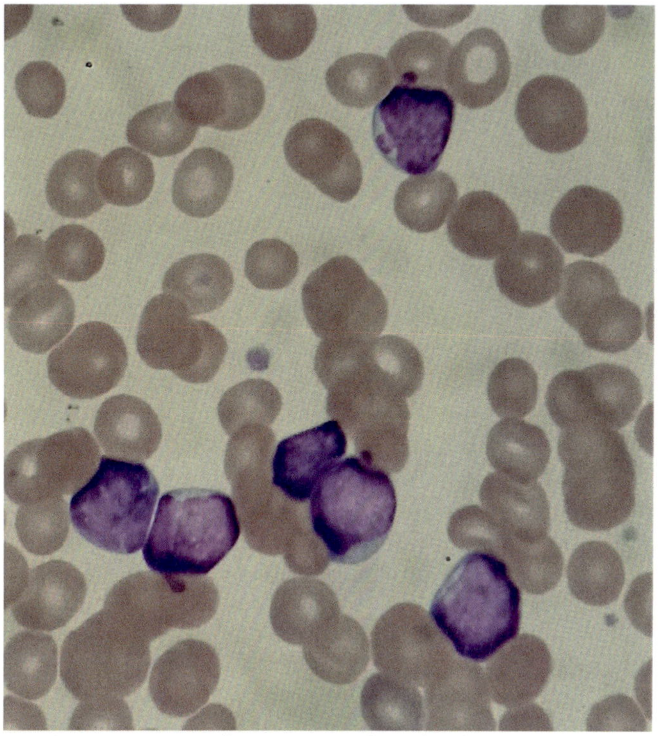

FIGURE 18.1.128 - Peripheral Blood Smear Showing Immature Lymphoblasts

V. Acute Lymphoblastic Leukemia: Management
   A. Systemic chemotherapy
   B. Targeted chemotherapy administered to CNS (intrathecally) and testes

REVIEW QUESTIONS

1. A 4-year-old boy is brought to his primary care physician by his parents because of a swollen, red face and arms. The mother first noticed swelling and redness 1 week ago and these symptoms have progressively worsened. The patient also feels fatigue for the last 2 months. He has difficulty swallowing the solid food. The physical exam shows hepatosplenomegaly, generalized lymphadenopathy, and diffuse petechiae. Peripheral blood smear shows immature lymphocytes. The tissue specimen obtained by bone marrow aspiration shows positivity for terminal deoxynucleotidyl transferase. What is the most likely cell of origin of this patient's condition?
    - **The most likely cell of origin is T cell.**
    - This patient presents with a swollen, red face and arms.
    - This is consistent with the diagnosis of superior vena cava syndrome.
    - He has difficulty swallowing the solid food suggesting esophageal compression.
    - Additionally, he has fatigue, hepatosplenomegaly, generalized lymphadenopathy, and diffuse petechiae.
    - Blood smear shows immature lymphocytes, and the tissue specimen is positive for terminal deoxynucleotidyl transferase.
    - This is a classic description of acute lymphoblastic leukemia.
    - Considering that this patient has signs of mediastinal infiltration such as superior vena cava syndrome and esophageal compression, the most likely cell of origin is T cell.

2. A 7-year-old girl is brought to her primary care physician by her father because of severe fatigue for the past week. The patient feels sleepy right after coming home from school and too tired to do her homework. The patient reports frequent nosebleeds without trauma. She is at the 5th percentile for her height and weight. Previous charts report that she was at the 25th percentile for both parameters 1 year ago. Vital signs are unremarkable. Physical examination shows generalized lymphadenopathy with mobile, non-tender lymph nodes. The liver is palpable 4 cm below the right costal margin. There are non-blanchable, nonpalpable purple spots all over her body. Which of the following is the best initial test in the diagnosis of this patient?

    A. Complete blood count with WBC differential
    B. Peripheral blood smear
    C. Bone marrow biopsy
    D. Genetic testing for *t(12;21)*

    - **The correct answer is option A.**
    - This patient presents with severe fatigue, suggesting anemia.
    - She also reports frequent nosebleeds without trauma, indicating possible thrombocytopenia.
    - Thrombocytopenia is further supported by non-blanchable, nonpalpable purple spots over her body that are petechiae.
    - Her growth charts suggest failure to thrive as her growth parameters have fallen below the normal range.
    - Hepatomegaly and generalized lymphadenopathy with mobile, non-tender lymph nodes, together with the other findings, point towards the diagnosis of leukemia.
    - The most common type of leukemia in this age is acute lymphoblastic leukemia.
    - The best initial test in the patient with suspected leukemia is a complete blood count with white blood cell (WBC) differential.
    - A complete blood count will likely show absolute lymphocytosis, anemia, and thrombocytopenia in this case.
    - Option B is incorrect because although a peripheral blood smear would be performed later to check for immature lymphoblasts, the number of malignant leukocytes must first be checked with a complete blood count.
    - Option C is incorrect because bone marrow biopsy is an invasive procedure, and it is the confirmatory, rather than initial, test for the patient with suspected leukemia.
    - Option D is incorrect because genetic testing is not cost-effective as an initial test, and not all patients with acute lymphoblastic leukemia have a *12;21* translocation.

Pediatrics | Section 32: Neuroblastoma and Wilms Tumor

I. Neuroblastoma: General Features
   A. Neuroendocrine tumor most commonly in children < 4 years of age
   B. Location
      1. Adrenal medulla (most common)
      2. Can occur anywhere along the sympathetic chain

II. Neuroblastoma: Pathophysiology
   A. Amine precursor uptake decarboxylase (APUD) tumor
   B. Derived from neural crest cells
   C. Overexpression of *N-myc* oncogene (codes for transcription factor)
   D. Produces catecholamines (norepinephrine, epinephrine, dopamine)

III. Neuroblastoma: Clinical Presentation
   A. Firm, irregular flank mass crossing the midline (vs. Wilms tumor)
   B. Normotensive (catecholamines rapidly degraded)
   C. Opsoclonus-myoclonus syndrome ("dancing eyes-dancing feet")

IV. Neuroblastoma: Diagnosis
   A. Urine vanillylmandelic acid (VMA) and homovanillic acid (HVA)
   B. CT of abdomen and pelvis
   C. Biopsy
      1. Homer-Wright rosettes (neuroblasts surrounding central lumen); also seen in medulloblastoma
      2. Bombesin and neuron-specific enolase positive

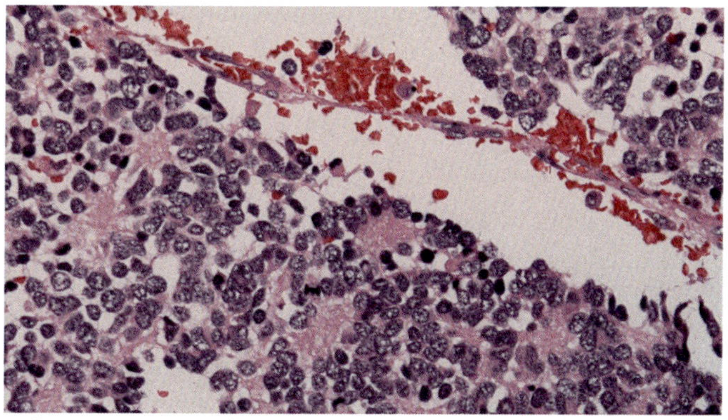

FIGURE 18.1.129 - Biopsy Showing Homer-Wright Rosettes

V. Neuroblastoma: Management
   A. Chemotherapy, radiotherapy, or surgery depending on the stage of the tumor and risks for complication

VI. Wilms Tumor: General Features
   A. Most common in children 2 - 4 years
   B. Tumor of immature renal parenchyma (nephroblastoma)

VII. Wilms Tumor: Genetic Abnormalities
   A. Genetic abnormalities
      1. Loss-of-function mutation in *WT1* or *WT2* genes on chromosome 11; can be associated with several genetic syndromes

VIII. Wilms Tumor: Clinical Presentation
   A. Smooth, regular flank mass not crossing the midline (vs. neuroblastoma)
   B. Hematuria and hypertension

IX. Wilms Tumor: WAGR Complex
   A. *WT1* deletion on chromosome 11
   B. **W**ilms tumor
   C. **A**niridia (no iris)
   D. **G**enitourinary malformations
   E. **R**ange of developmental delay

X. Wilms Tumor: Denys-Drash Syndrome
   A. *WT1* mutation rather than deletion
   B. Wilms tumor
   C. **D**iffuse mesangial sclerosis with early-onset nephrotic syndrome
   D. Gonadal **D**ysgenesis (46, XY DSD)

XI. Wilm Tumor: Beckwith-Wiedemann Syndrome
   A. *WT2* mutation
   B. Wilms tumor
   C. Organomegaly
   D. Macroglossia
   E. Hemihyperplasia of body
   F. Omphalocele

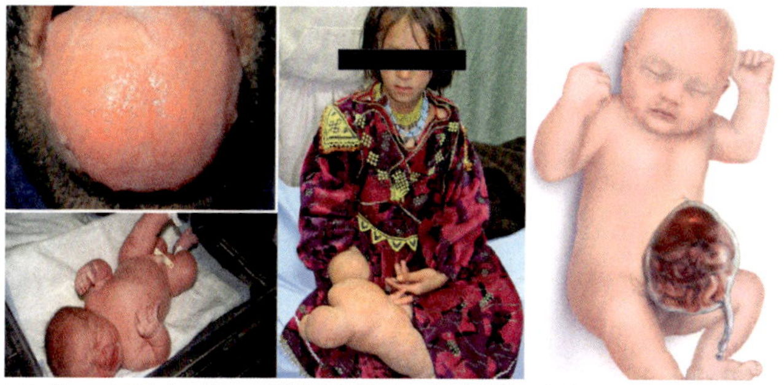

FIGURE 18.1.130 - Clinical Features of Beckwith-Wiedemann Syndrome

XII. Wilms Tumor: Diagnosis and Management
   A. Diagnosis
      1. Abdominal ultrasound (preferred) or CT scan
      2. Chest CT scan to look for pulmonary metastasis
      3. Biopsy
   B. Management
      1. Surgical excision
      2. Chemotherapy or radiotherapy

REVIEW QUESTIONS

1. A 3-year-old girl is brought to her primary care physician by her parents because of a right-sided flank mass they noticed 4 days ago during her bath. Her parents have also noticed that she moves her eyes back and forth and she has a constant urge to move her feet. Physical examination shows a right-sided flank mass that crosses the midline. The abdominal ultrasound shows a right adrenal mass. What is most likely to be found on the biopsy of this patient's flank mass?
    - **The biopsy of this patient's flank mass will likely show Homer-Wright rosettes.**
    - This patient has a right adrenal mass that crosses the midline.
    - Additionally, she moves her eyes back and forth, and she has a constant urge to move her feet.
    - This description is consistent with opsoclonus-myoclonus syndrome, also known as "dancing eyes-dancing feet."
    - The most likely diagnosis in this patient is neuroblastoma.
    - Biopsy of neuroblastoma usually shows Homer-Wright rosettes, the neuroblasts surrounding the central eosinophilic lumen.

2. A 3-year-old boy is brought to his primary care physician by his parents because of a left-sided flank mass. The mass was first noticed several days ago by his mother when she was bathing him. Physical examination shows a left mass that does not cross the midline. He has periorbital and peripheral edema. External genitalia is severely undervirilized. Urinalysis is significant for 4+ proteinuria. What is the most likely morphological change in renal tissue that best explains this patient's urinalysis findings?
    - **The morphological change in renal tissue that best explains this patient's nephrotic syndrome is diffuse mesangial sclerosis**
    - This patient presents with a left-sided flank mass that does not cross the midline.
    - This presentation likely suggests Wilms tumor.
    - His external genitalia are severely undervirilized indicating that he has *46, XY* disorder of sex development.
    - Finally, his urinalysis is significant for 4+ proteinuria, and the patient has periorbital and peripheral edema.
    - These latter clues indicate the presence of nephrotic syndrome.
    - The triad of Wilms tumor, gonadal dysgenesis, and an early-onset nephrotic syndrome is characteristic of Denys-Drash syndrome.

Pediatrics | Section 33: Osteosarcoma and Ewing Sarcoma

I. Osteosarcoma: General Features
   A. Malignant osteoblast tumor
      1. 1° osteosarcoma: males < 20 years (most common cohort)
      2. 2° osteosarcoma: elderly with predisposing factors (e.g. bone infarcts, Paget disease of the bone, radiation)
   B. Hereditary osteosarcoma
      1. Li-Fraumeni syndrome also known as SBLA (TP53 gene mutation)
      2. Familial retinoblastoma (RB1 gene mutation)

II. Osteosarcoma: Clinical Presentation
   A. Localized bone pain
   B. Enlarging bone mass most commonly in the distal femoral metaphysis
   C. Pathological fractures

III. Osteosarcoma: Diagnosis
   A. Bone X-ray: Codman triangle; "sunburst" pattern of bone
   B. Biopsy: pleomorphic osteoid-producing cells

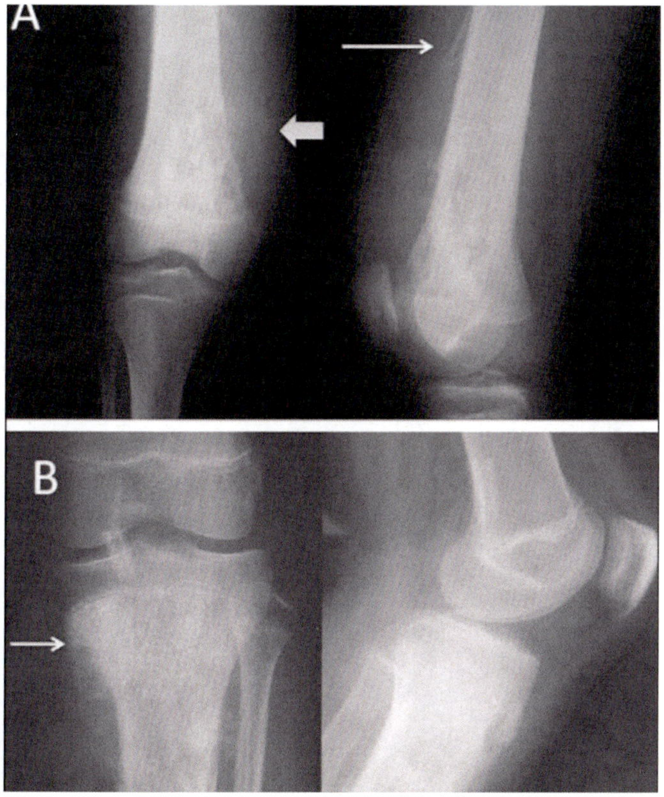

FIGURE 18.1.131 - X-ray Knee Showing Codman Triangle and Sunburst Pattern in Osteosarcoma

IV. Osteosarcoma: Management
   A. Surgery, chemotherapy
   B. 1° osteosarcoma - better prognosis
   C. 2° osteosarcoma - worse prognosis

V. Ewing Sarcoma: General Features
   A. Common in white males < 15 years of age
   B. Neuroectodermal tumor
   C. Location
      1. Diaphysis of long bones (commonly femur)
      2. Pelvic flat bones

VI. Ewing Sarcoma: Diagnosis
   A. Bone X-ray: "onion skin" periosteal reaction
   B. Biopsy: anaplastic small blue cells
   C. Cytogenetic testing: t(11;22) - EWS-FLI1 fusion protein to differentiate from lymphoma and chronic osteomyelitis

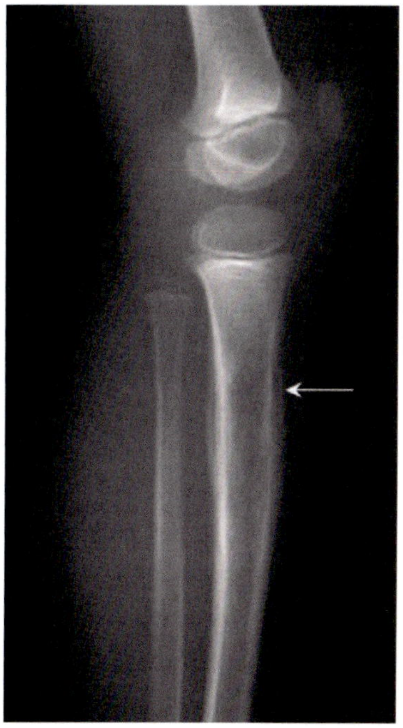

FIGURE 18.1.132 - X-ray Knee Showing "Onion Skin" Periosteal Reaction in Ewing Sarcoma

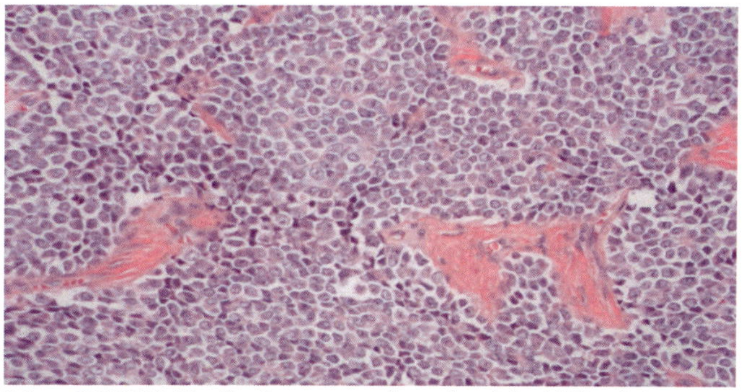

FIGURE 18.1.133 - Biopsy Showing Anaplastic Blue Cells in Ewing Sarcoma

VII. Ewing Sarcoma: Management
   A. Surgery
   B. Chemotherapy

REVIEW QUESTIONS

1. A 12-year-old boy is brought to his primary care physician because of pain in his right thigh. He first noticed the pain 6 months ago, and it has progressively worsened. He cannot bear weight on his right leg while walking anymore. Vital signs include a temperature of 38° C (100.4° F), blood pressure of 125/75 mmHg, heart rate of 91 beats/min, and respiratory rate of 15 breaths/min. Physical examination shows focal tenderness on the right anterior thigh. An X-ray of the right lower extremity shows a mass in the femoral diaphysis with a surrounding concentric periosteal reaction. A biopsy of the mass shows small blue cells. Which of the following is the next best step in the management?

    A. Cytogenetic analysis for t(11;22)
    B. Amputation of the affected extremity
    C. Chemotherapy
    D. IV antibiotic therapy

- **The correct answer is option A.**
- This patient presents with right thigh pain and tenderness, inability to bear weight on the ipsilateral leg, and low-grade fever.
- X-ray of the right lower extremity shows a mass in the femoral diaphysis with the surrounding concentric periosteal reaction.
- This description likely suggests an "onion skin" periosteal reaction.
- A biopsy of the mass shows small blue cells.
- The differential diagnosis of this patient's condition is either Ewing sarcoma, lymphoma metastatic to bone, or chronic osteomyelitis with lymphocytic infiltration.
- This translocation is present in Ewing sarcoma but absent in lymphoma and chronic osteomyelitis.
- Options B, amputation of the affected extremity, and option C, chemotherapy, are incorrect because although they are commonly used in the management of patients with Ewing sarcoma, we first need to confirm that this patient truly has Ewing sarcoma.
- Option D, IV antibiotic therapy, is incorrect because although it is used in chronic osteomyelitis, we first need to find out the exact cause of this patient's condition.

I. Cerebral Palsy: Definition
   A. Group of non-hereditary and non-progressive disorders that involve permanent motor dysfunction including abnormal tone, posture, and/or movement

II. Cerebral Palsy: Etiology
   A. Etiology unknown
   B. Prenatal or perinatal insult to the brain

III. Cerebral Palsy: Risk Factors
   A. Prematurity (e.g. intraventricular hemorrhage, periventricular leukomalacia)
   B. IUGR
   C. Perinatal hypoxic-ischemic injury
   D. Intrauterine infection (e.g. TORCHES)
   E. Trauma
   F. Tobacco use, alcohol

IV. Cerebral Palsy: Classification
   A. Spastic (most common)
      1. Diplegic, hemiplegic, quadriplegic
      2. Spasticity (toe-walking), hyperreflexia (↑ DTR), positive babinski sign; equinovarus deformity of feet
   B. Nonspastic
      1. Dyskinetic: involuntary movements (dystonia, athetosis, chorea)
      2. Ataxic: lack of coordination

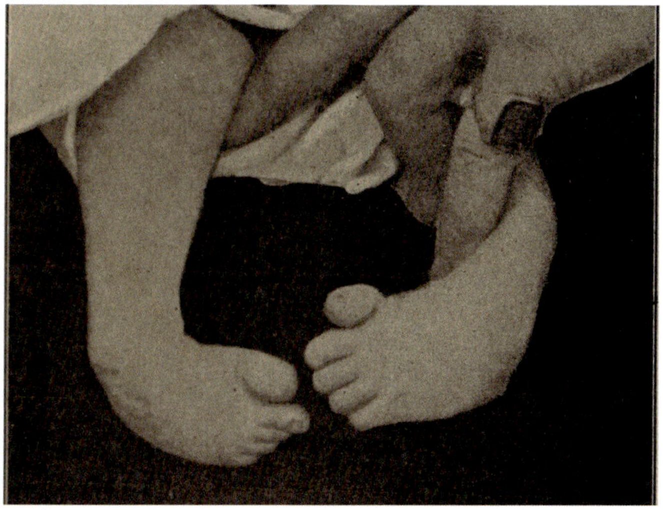

https://www.flickr.com/photos/internetarchivebookimages/14764736742/sizes/o/

FIGURE 18.1.134 - Equinovarus Deformity

V. Cerebral Palsy: Clinical Features
   A. Delayed achievement of motor milestones
   B. Gait abnormalities: toe walking, scissoring of legs, commando crawl
   C. Joint contractures
   D. Intellectual disability
   E. Swallowing difficulties; drooling
   F. Abnormal speech
   G. Comorbidities: epilepsy, scoliosis, strabismus

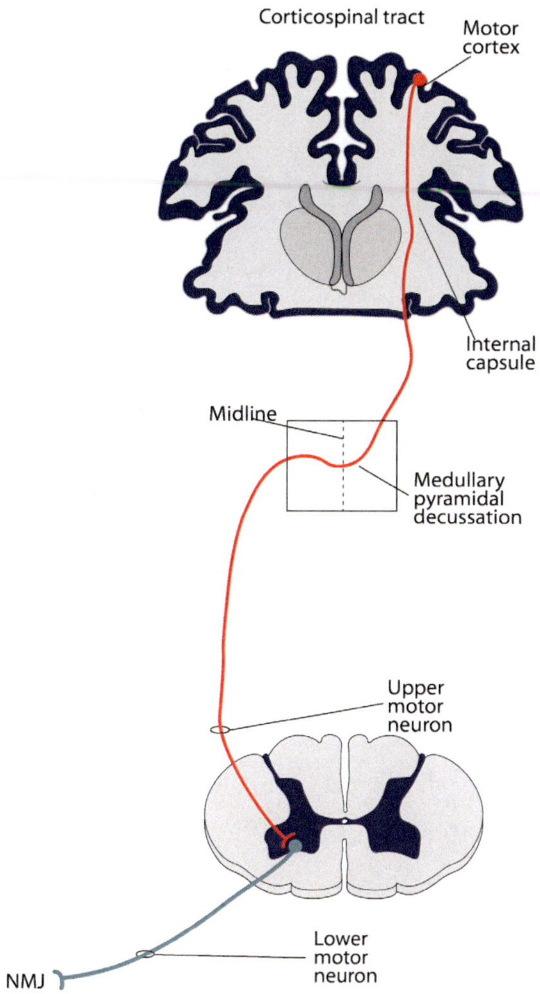

FIGURE 18.1.135 - Corticospinal Tract

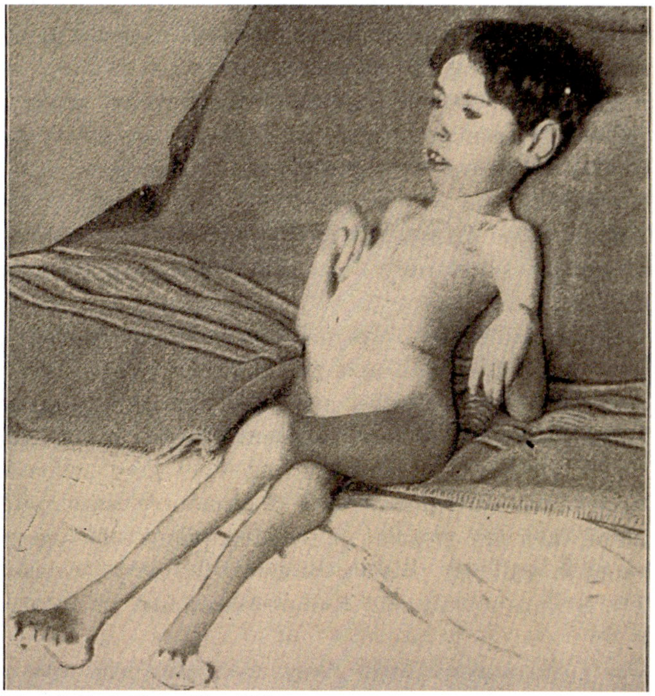

Internet Archive Book Images / No restrictions

FIGURE 18.1.136 - Spastic Cerebral Palsy

VI. Cerebral Palsy: Diagnosis
   A. Mainly clinical diagnosis
   B. Imaging: structural causes (e.g. intraventricular hemorrhage, periventricular leukomalacia)
      1. Cranial ultrasound
      2. MRI

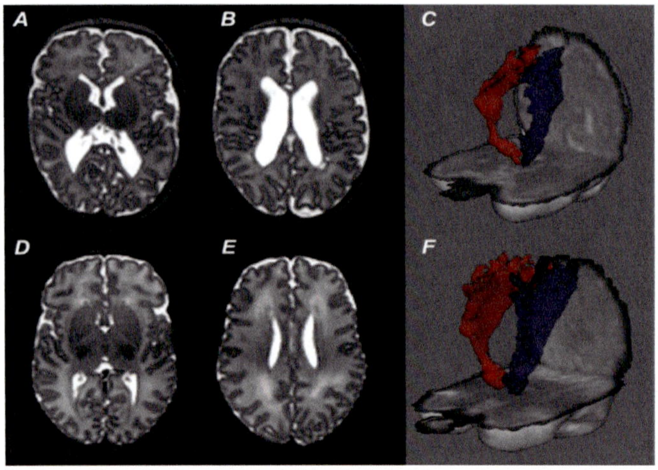

FIGURE 18.1.137 - MRI of the Brain: Cystic Periventricular Malacia

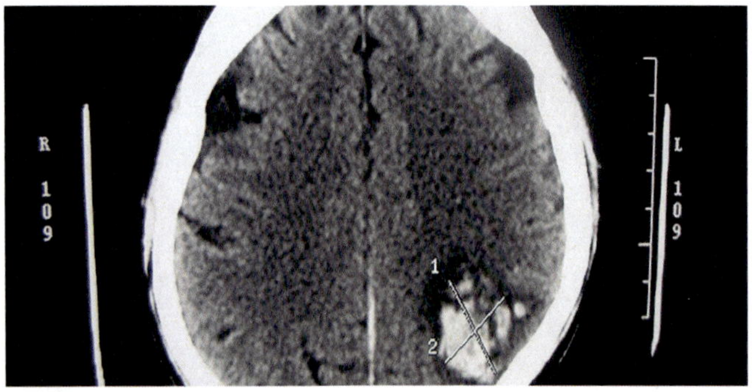

FIGURE 18.1.139 - CT Scan of the Head: Intracerebral Hemorrhage

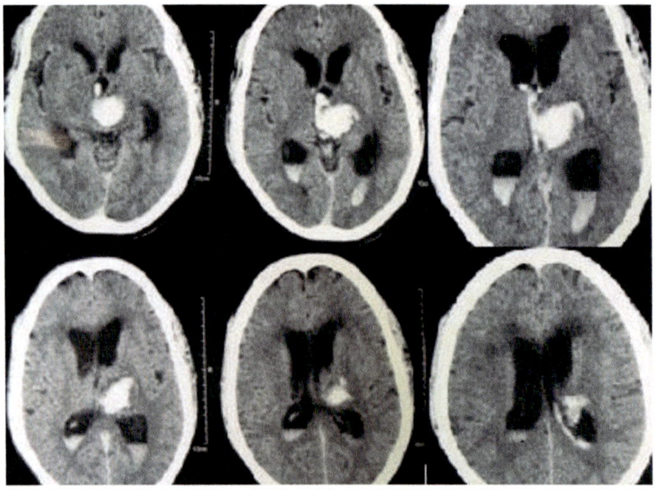

FIGURE 18.1.140 - CT Scan of the Head: Intraventricular Hemorrhage

VII. Cerebral Palsy: Management
   A. No cure
   B. Multidisciplinary approach
      1. Special education
      2. Physical therapy
      3. Antispastic medications: baclofen pumps, botulinum toxin
      4. Surgical release of contractures
      5. Magnesium sulfate: for mothers at risk of premature delivery

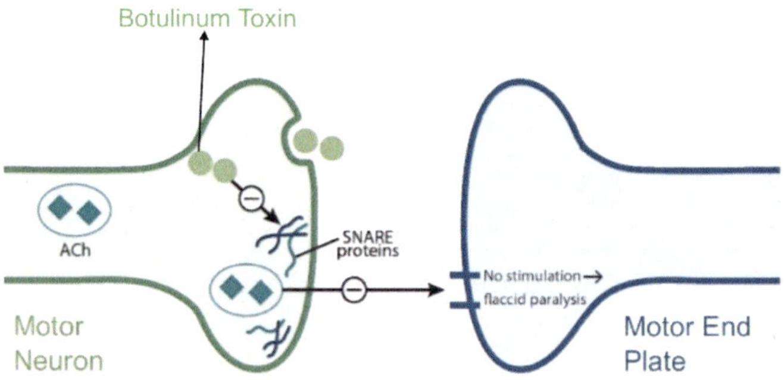

FIGURE 18.1.141 - Botulinum Toxin

VIII. Infantile Hypotonia: Definition
   A. Decreased muscle tone
   B. Sign of CNS, primary neuromuscular, or genetic disorder

IX. Infantile Hypotonia: Etiology
   A. Genetic syndromes: Down syndrome, Prader-Willi syndrome
   B. Inborn errors of metabolism: glycogen storage diseases, Tay-Sachs disease
   C. Infections: botulism
   D. Neuromuscular disorders: spinal muscular atrophy, myotonic dystrophy
   E. Endocrine abnormalities: congenital hypothyroidism, hypoglycemia

X. Infantile Hypotonia: Diagnosis
   A. Obstetric and perinatal history
   B. General appearance: dysmorphic features, congenital defects
      1. Frog-like position, decreased spontaneous activity, decreased muscle tone
   C. Complete neurologic examination
   D. Management depends on the etiology

REVIEW QUESTIONS

1. An 18-month-old girl is brought to her primary care physician by her mother because of her inability to walk normally. Physical examination shows toe-walking and scissoring of the legs. Deep tendon reflexes are hyperactive, and Babinski reflex is positive bilaterally. She was born at 33 weeks gestation due to preterm prelabor rupture of membranes. What is the optimal management of this patient's condition?

    - **The optimal management of this patient's condition is a multidisciplinary approach, including special education, physical therapy, antispastic medications, and surgery for contractures.**
    - This 18-month-old girl presents with toe-walking and scissoring of the legs. This finding indicates hypertonia in the lower extremities.
    - Deep tendon reflexes are hyperactive, and the Babinski reflex is positive bilaterally. These clues suggest upper motor neuron damage.
    - Given all these findings and the fact that she was born preterm at 33 weeks gestation, she likely has spastic cerebral palsy.

2. A 6-month-old boy is brought to his primary care physician by his parents because of increased sleepiness and weakness for the past week. The infant has a weak cry. His mother says she has recently been giving him honey to "grow healthier." Physical examination shows a lethargic infant with hypotonic extremities and 1+ reflexes. What is the most likely diagnosis?

    - **The most likely diagnosis is infantile botulism.**
    - This infant presents with increased sleepiness and weakness.
    - Physical examination shows hypotonic extremities and 1+ reflexes.
    - Given that the mother has been giving him honey, there is a high suspicion for infantile botulism.
    - This is because the *Clostridium botulinum* spores are ingested with honey and germinate in the gastrointestinal tract.
    - Botulism typically causes a descending paralysis with hypotonia and hyporeflexia.

3. A 12-month-old boy is brought to his primary care physician because of a failure to reach developmental milestones. He still has not learned to sit or crawl. He babbles but does not make concrete sounds. He also has feeding problems and often chokes during feeding. His elbows and knees are flexed. Physical examination shows spasticity and increased tone in the upper and lower extremities. He also has slight strabismus. An MRI of the brain reveals periventricular leukomalacia. Which of the following is the most important risk factor for the development of this condition?

    A. Congenital CMV infection
    B. Congenital toxoplasmosis infection
    C. Maternal alcohol during pregnancy
    D. Premature birth

    - **The correct answer is option D.**
    - This 12-month-old boy is brought in because he wasn't reaching his developmental milestones.
    - He has upper motor neuron signs such as spasticity and increased tone.
    - Babies should be able to sit unsupported by the age of 7-9 months and start to crawl by the age of 9 months. By the age of 12 months, babies should be able to say a few words like "mama and dada" distinctly, which this child isn't at this time.
    - Brain MRI reveals periventricular leukomalacia, which is frequently present in patients with cerebral palsy.
    - All these features make spastic cerebral palsy the most likely diagnosis.
    - The most important risk factors for developing cerebral palsy are premature birth and low birth weight.
    - Option A is incorrect because although congenital CMV infection increases the risk of CP, a brain MRI would show periventricular calcifications, not periventricular leukomalacia. Furthermore, features of congenital CMV infection, such as a skin rash, seizures, and microcephaly, are absent in this patient.
    - Option B is incorrect because although congenital toxoplasmosis increases the risk of CP, a brain MRI would show intracranial calcifications instead. Also, features of congenital toxoplasmosis infection, such as microcephaly, hydrocephalus, and chorioretinitis, are all absent in this patient.
    - Option C is incorrect because although maternal alcohol during pregnancy increases the risk of CP, features of fetal alcohol syndrome such as a small head, short nose, and thin upper lip are absent in this patient.

Pediatrics | Section 35: MSK Disorders - Hip Conditions

I. Legg-Calvé-Perthes Disease
   A. Idiopathic avascular necrosis of the femoral head
   B. Affects children (age 4-10 years); peak incidence at age 5-7 years
   C. Boys > girls
   D. Etiology: idiopathic, familial; can be due to hemophilia or repetitive trauma
   E. Clinical features: insidious onset hip pain projecting to the knee, limp, antalgic gait; unilateral or bilateral; ↓ ROM
   F. Physical examination: ↑ pain and limited ROM on internal rotation and abduction; atrophy of thigh muscles
   G. Diagnosis: x-ray may be normal (early stages), fragmentation and sclerosis of the femoral head (late changes); MRI if the x-ray is inconclusive
   H. Differential diagnosis: transient synovitis which occurs after a viral infection; resolves in 1-4 weeks
   I. Management
      1. Conservative with rest, NSAIDs, bracing, avoid weight-bearing exercises
      2. Surgery with femoral osteotomy: age ≥ 6 years, extensive damage where the femoral head is not contained in the acetabulum
   J. Complications include early-onset osteoarthritis
   K. Prognosis: depends on the age of onset and degree of femoral involvement
      1. Early onset (< 6-8 years) is associated with a better prognosis

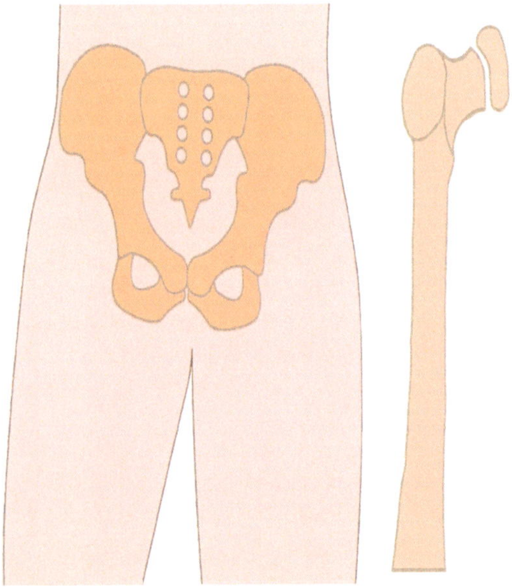

FIGURE 18.1.142 - Subluxation and Displacement of Femoral Head After Necrosis

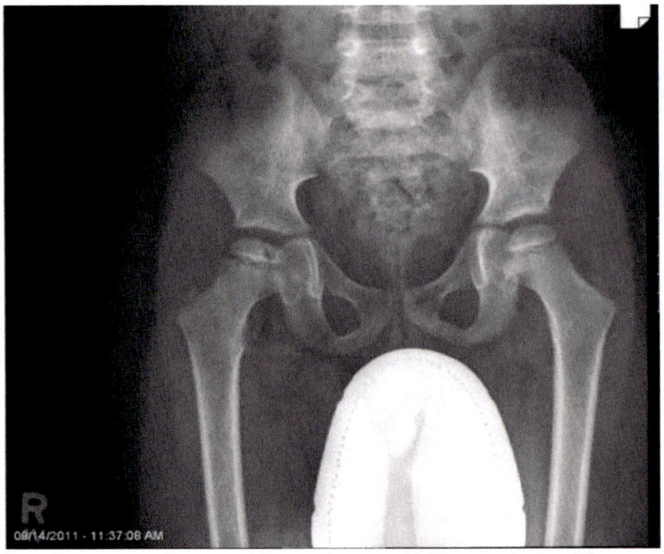

FIGURE 18.1.143 - Pelvic X-Ray Showing Flattening of Both Femoral Heads

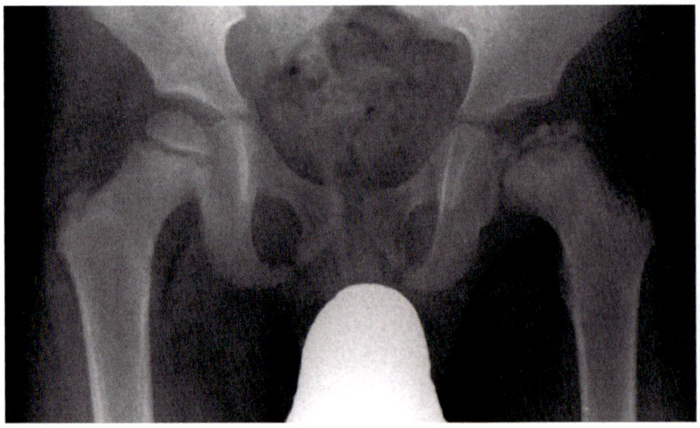

FIGURE 18.1.144 - Pelvic X-Ray Showing Necrosis and Fragmentation of the left Femoral Head

II. Slipped Capital Femoral Epiphysis (SCFE)
   A. A hip disorder characterized by displacement of the femoral head at the proximal growth plate relative to the femoral neck
   B. Affects adolescent males 10-16 years (↑ growth)
   C. Due to weakening of the epiphyseal plate and increased shearing
   D. Risk factors include positive family history, obesity, trauma, endocrine disorders, renal failure, and history of radiation
   E. Clinical features: pain and gait disturbance
      1. Dull, aching hip, groin, or knee pain; increases with physical activity; acute or chronic; limp
   F. Physical exam
      1. ↓ ROM, decreased internal rotation and abduction; limb shortening, inability to bear weight
      2. Patients hold the hip in external rotation

G. Diagnosis
    1. X-ray, ultrasound, MRI
    2. Posterior and inferior displacement of the femoral head and widened joint space; both hips should be assessed
H. Management
    1. Urgent surgical internal fixation
    2. Avoid weight-bearing
I. Follow-up: risk of involvement of the other hip
J. Complications: avascular necrosis of the femoral head, early-onset hip osteoarthritis

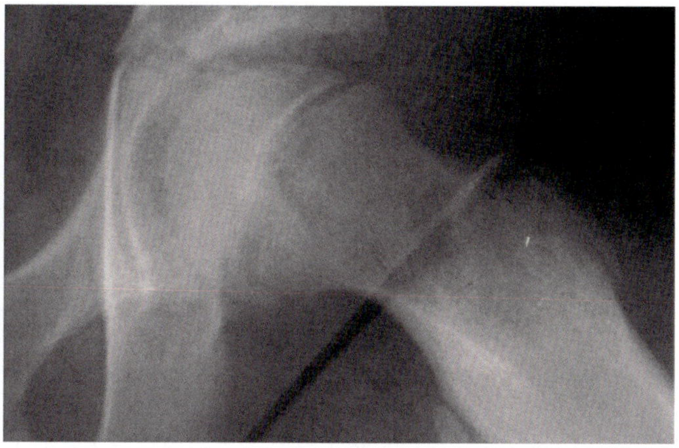

Mikir at English Wikipedia, Public domain, via Wikimedia Commons

FIGURE 18.1.145 - X-Ray of the Hip Joint

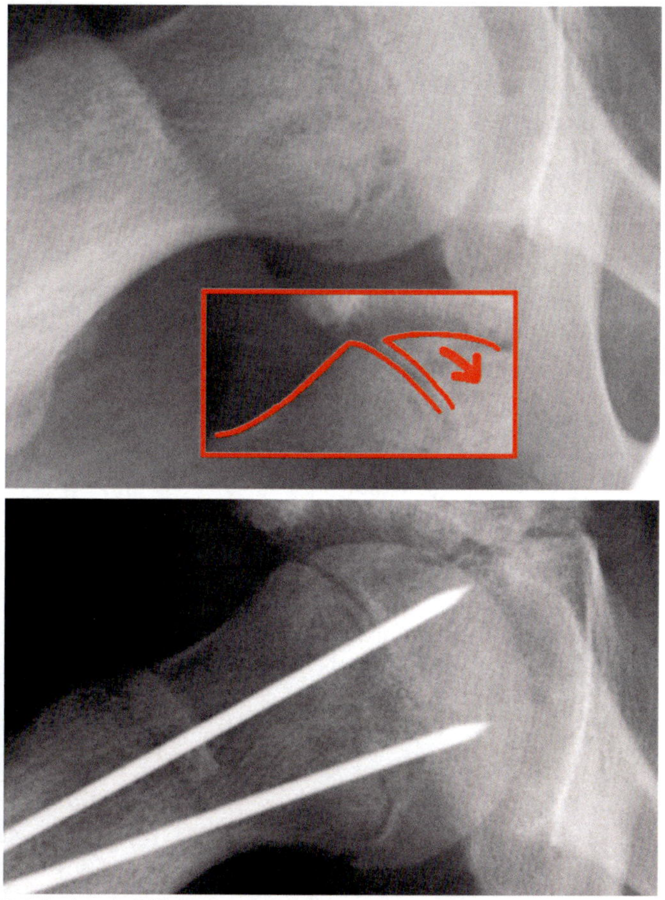

Dr. Jochen Lengerke, Public domain, via Wikimedia Commons

FIGURE 18.1.146 - X-Ray Showing Slipped Capital Femoral Epiphysis, Before and After Surgical Intervention

III. Developmental Dysplasia of Hip
    A. Subluxation or dislocation of the femoral head, and/or dysplasia of the acetabulum
    B. Unknown etiology
    C. Risk factors
        1. Breech positioning
        2. Positive family history
        3. Female sex, first born child
    D. Clinical features
        1. Click or clunk in the hip
            a) When the hip is flexed and abducted while applying anterior force (Ortolani sign)
            b) When the hip is flexed and adducted while applying posterior force (Barlow sign)
            c) Can be detected in patients < 6 months of age
    E. Clinical features
        1. Galeazzi sign, difficulty in hip abduction
        2. Hip pain, trendelenburg gait
        3. Asymmetrical folds of thigh, gluteal and inguinal regions; limb length discrepancy (absent in bilateral conditions)
    F. Diagnosis
        1. Screening physical examination on every well visit <6 months
        2. Age < 4 months: hip ultrasound
        3. Age > 4 months: pelvic x-ray
        4. Imaging helps confirm the diagnosis and assess acetabular development
    G. Treatment
        1. Pavlik harness: < 6 months; splint to hold the hip in flexion and abduction position
        2. Closed reduction with hip spica cast: 6-18 months
        3. Open reduction with hip splice cast: > 18 months; pelvic or femoral osteotomy

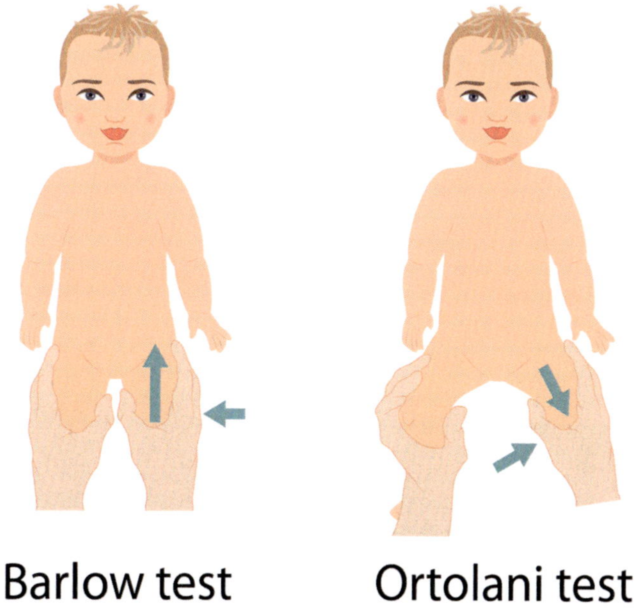

FIGURE 18.1.118 - Barlow & Ortolani Tests

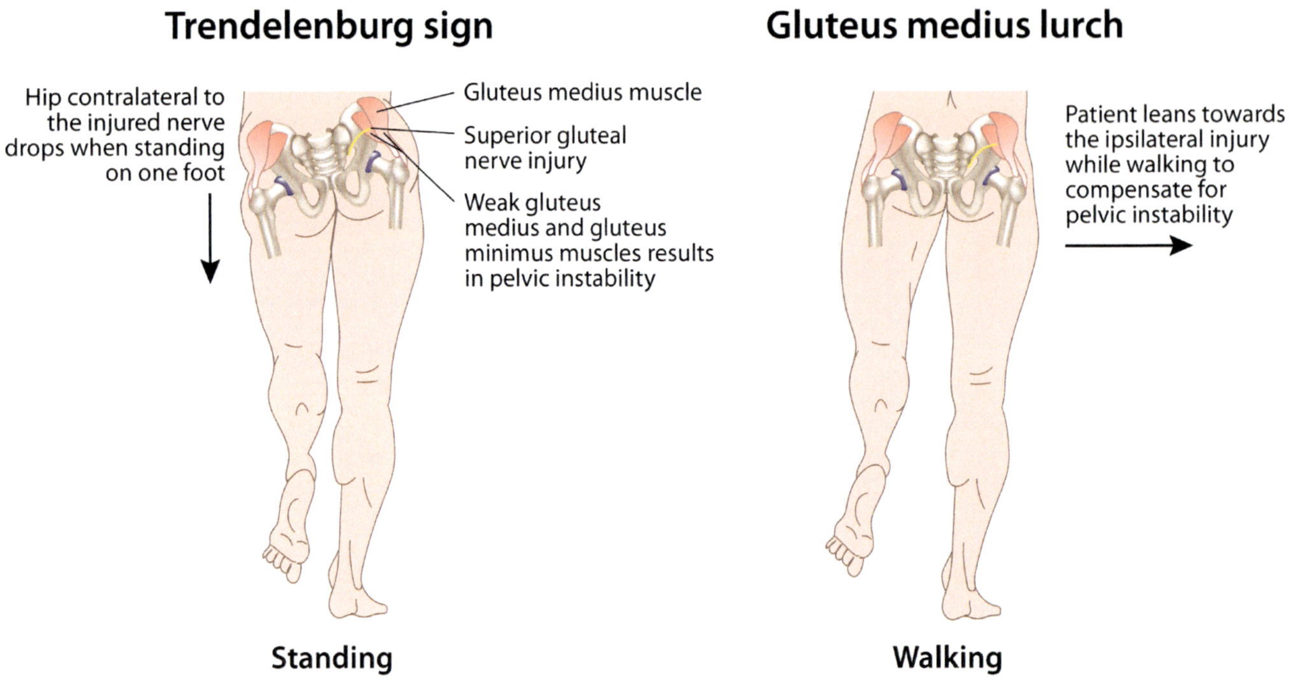

FIGURE 18.1.147 - Trendelenburg Gait

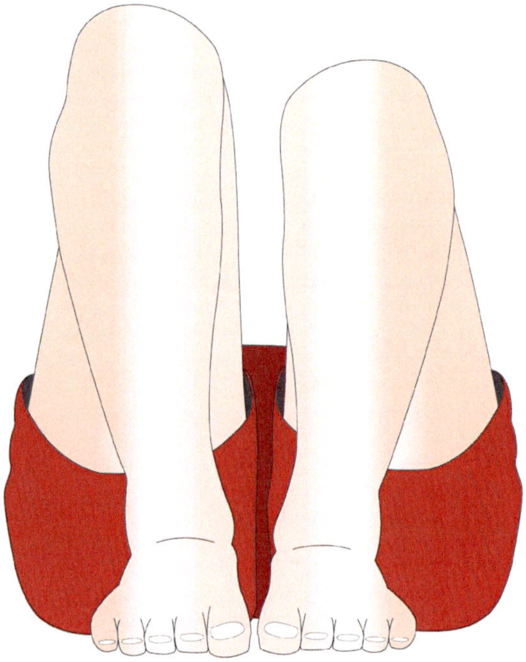

FIGURE 18.1.119 - Galeazzi Sign

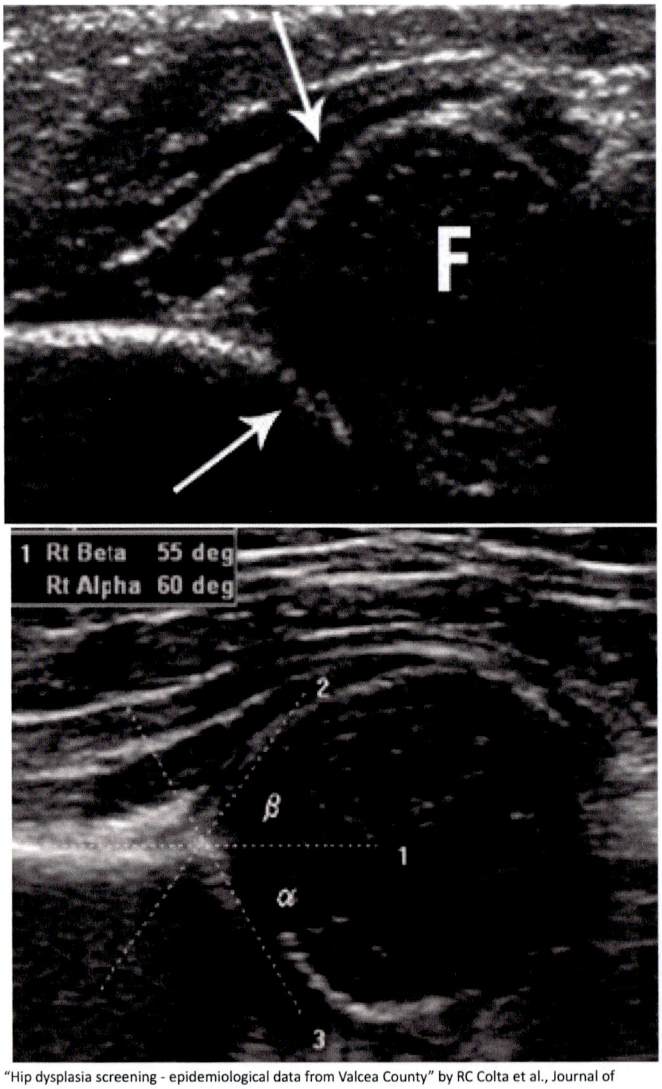

FIGURE 18.1.148 - Normal Hip Ultrasound in an Infant

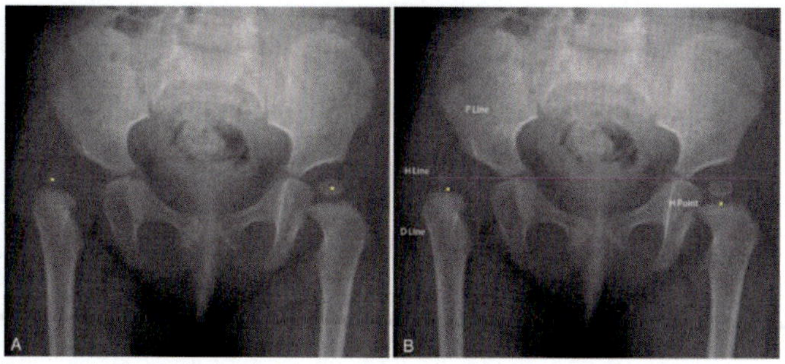

"Retrospective observational study comparing the international hip dysplasia institute classification with the Tonnis classification of developmental dysplasia of the hip" by Mingyuan Miao et al., Medicine is licensed under CC BY 4.0

FIGURE 18.1.149 - Pelvic X-Ray Showing Developmental Dysplasia of the Right Hip

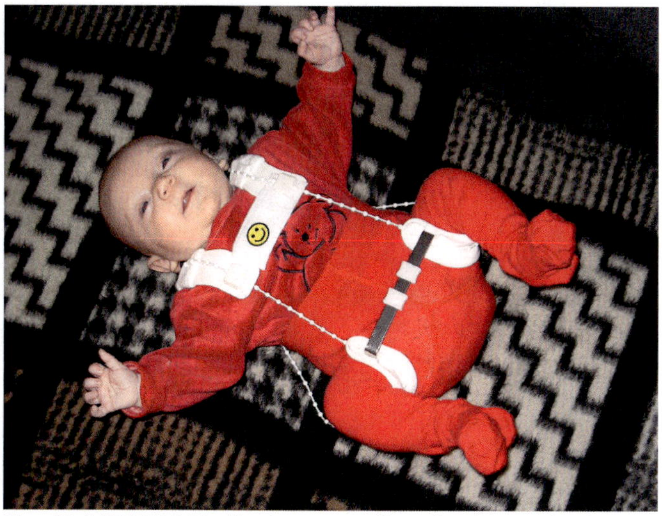

Thiemo Schuff, CC BY-SA 3.0 <https://creativecommons.org/licenses/by-sa/3.0>, via Wikimedia Commons

FIGURE 18.1.150 - Baby Wearing Pavlik Harness

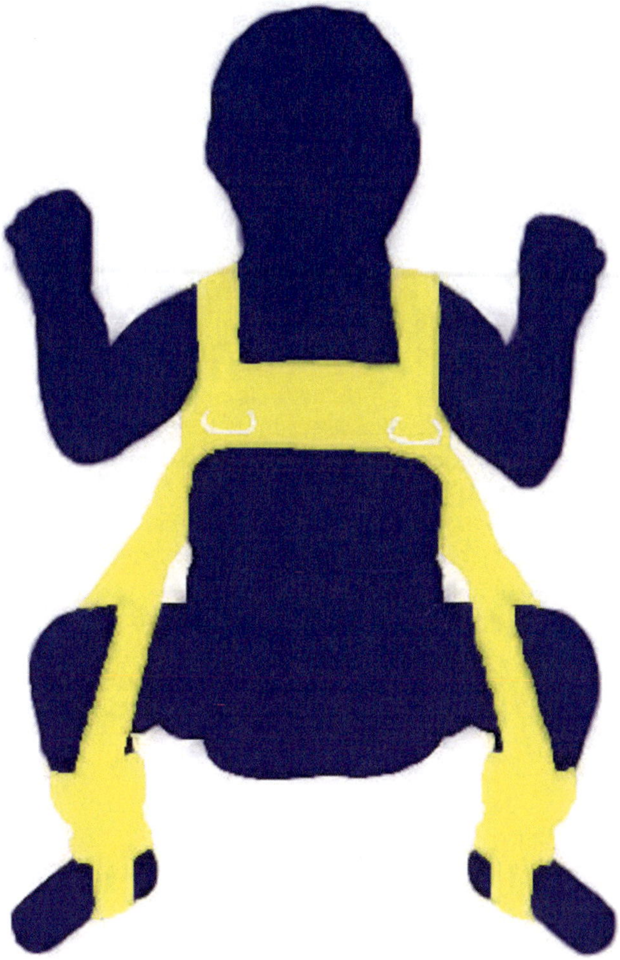

Londenp, CC BY-SA 3.0 <http://creativecommons.org/licenses/by-sa/3.0/>, via Wikimedia Commons

FIGURE 18.1.151 - Diagram of Baby Wearing a Pavlik Harness

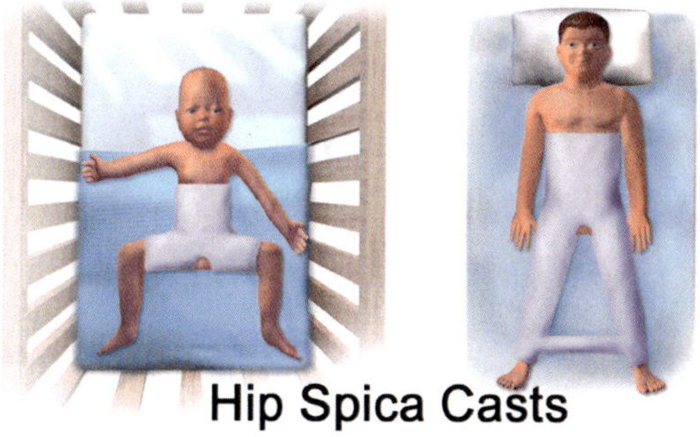

BruceBlaus, CC BY-SA 4.0 <https://creativecommons.org/licenses/by-sa/4.0>, via Wikimedia Commons

FIGURE 18.1.152 - Hip Spica Cast Treatment

REVIEW QUESTIONS

1. A 6-year-old boy is brought to his primary care physician by his parents because of insidious limping and hip pain for the past 4 months. He has recently refused to play with other children in the yard due to hip pain. The physical examination shows pain exacerbation upon internal rotation and abduction of his left hip. Pelvic X-ray shows flattened femoral epiphysis with hyperlucent areas. What is the most likely diagnosis in this patient?
   - **The most likely diagnosis in this patient is Legg-Calvé-Perthes disease.**
   - This boy presents with insidious limping and hip pain for the past 4 months.
   - The physical examination shows pain exacerbation upon internal rotation and abduction of his left hip.
   - His age, gender, and symptoms are all classic for Legg-Calve-Perthes disease.
   - Legg-Calvé-Perthes disease is confirmed by the pelvic X-ray findings of flattened femoral epiphysis with hyperlucent areas.

2. A 2-month-old girl is brought to her primary care physician by her parents because of a "shorter right leg". She was born at 39 weeks of gestation without prenatal or perinatal complications. An audible clunk is elicited by flexing and abducting the hip with applying anterior force or flexing and adducting the hip with applying posterior force. Hip ultrasound shows femoral head dislocated from the acetabular fossa. What is the best initial treatment option for this patient's condition?
   - **The best initial treatment option for the developmental dysplasia of the hip in patients less than 6 months of age is Pavlik harness.**
   - This 2-months-old girl presents with a "shorter right leg".
   - This phenomenon is referred to as leg length discrepancy.
   - An audible clunk is elicited by flexing and abducting the hip with applying anterior force or flexing and adducting the hip with applying posterior force.
   - These findings describe Ortolani and Barlow maneuvers, respectively.
   - Hip ultrasound shows femoral head dislocated from the acetabular fossa.
   - All of these clues are consistent with the diagnosis of developmental dysplasia of the hip.
   - Pavlik harness keeps both hips flexed and abducted so that femoral heads stay in the acetabular fossa.

3. A 14-year-old male is brought to his primary care physician by his mother because of right hip pain. His mother also adds that he has been walking abnormally. The physical exam shows an obese boy sitting in the office in no acute distress. The patient's right hip is noted to be shorter than the left and he is holding the hip in external rotation as he is examined. His vital signs show temperature of 99.7°F (37.6°C), heart rate of 70 beats/min, respiratory rate of 12 breaths/min, and blood pressure of 120/80 mmHg. His BMI is 33 Kg/m2. Based on this patient's most likely diagnosis, which of the following options is a potential complication of his condition?

   A. Rheumatoid arthritis
   B. Avascular necrosis
   C. Osteosarcoma
   D. Osteomyelitis

   - **The correct answer is B.**
   - A 14-year-old male presents due to right hip pain and an abnormal gait.
   - On physical exam, he is noted to be obese which is confirmed by the BMI of 33.
   - Additionally, his right hip is shorter than the left and he is holding it in external rotation.
   - Based on this presentation, the patient most likely has slipped capital femoral epiphysis aka SCFE.
   - Answer choice A is incorrect because early onset hip osteoarthritis is a potential complication of SCFE, but rheumatoid arthritis is not.
   - Answer choice C is incorrect because the risk of osteosarcoma is associated with retinoblastoma, not SCFE.
   - Answer choice D is incorrect because the risk of osteomyelitis is not associated with SCFE, but rather can be seen when an adjacent infection spreads to the bone in a diabetic.

Pediatrics | Section 36: MSK Disorders: Foot Deformities

I. Club Foot
   A. Also known as congenital talipes equinovarus
   B. Widely common congenital deformity
   C. Mostly due to dominance of posterior tibial muscle
   D. Cavus of midfoot: high-arched foot
   E. Adductus of forefoot: toes are turned inwards
   F. Varus of hindfoot: heel is turned inwards
   G. Equinus of hindfoot: abnormal plantar flexion of foot
   H. Diagnosis
      1. Clinical
      2. X-ray: parallelism of talus and calcaneus long axes
   I. Management
      1. Serial stretching, manipulation and casting (Ponseti method)
      2. Surgery: if above method fails; usually performed within 3 - 6 months of age

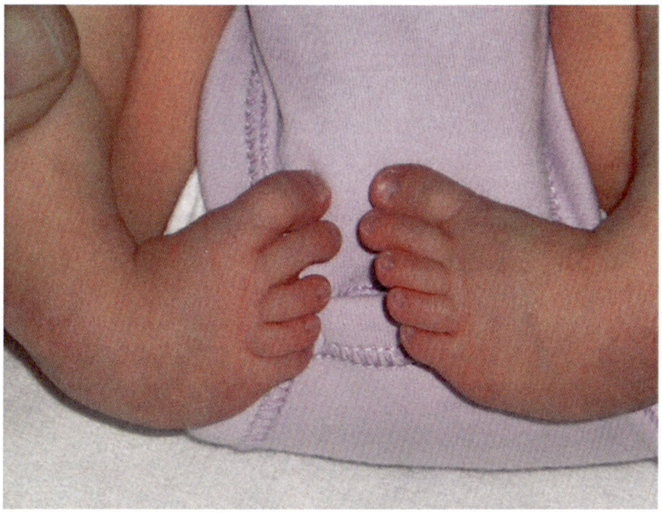

FIGURE 18.1.153 - Club Foot

II. Metatarsus Adductus
   A. Adduction of the forefoot with convex lateral border and concave medial border
   B. Hindfoot is in neutral position
   C. Mostly seen in the first born infants
   D. Can be associated with hip dysplasia
   E. Causes intoeing in children
   F. Diagnosis: clinical; imaging is not required
   G. Management
      1. Mostly spontaneous resolution
      2. Corrective shoes or cast required for special cases

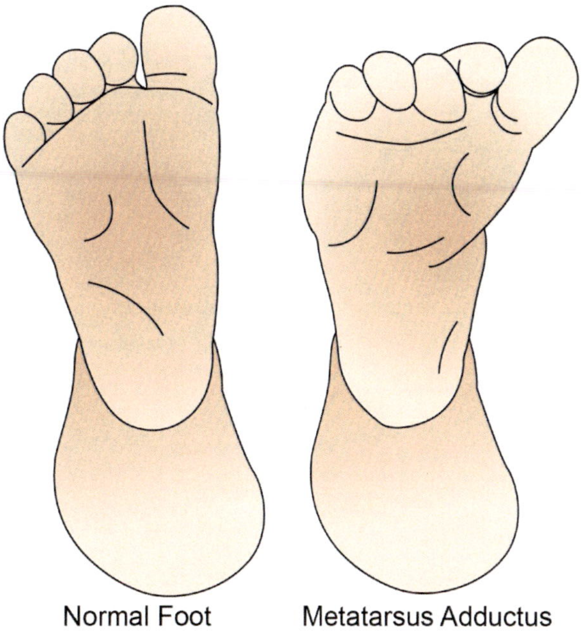

FIGURE 18.1.121 - Metatarsus Adductus

III. Pes Planus
   A. Flat foot; loss of medial longitudinal arch of foot
   B. Etiology
      1. Congenital: isolated or associated with neurological conditions
      2. Functional (e.g. dysfunction of posterior tibial tendon, trauma)
   C. Two types: rigid and flexible
      1. Flexible: intact arch during heel elevation or non weight-bearing
      2. Rigid: absent arch during weight-bearing and heel elevation
   D. Diagnosis
      1. Mainly clinical
      2. Lateral foot X-ray
   E. Management
      1. Serial casting after birth
      2. Surgery in case of failure

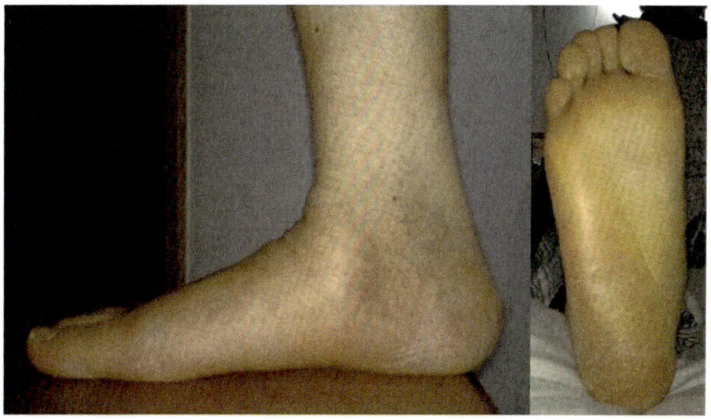

FIGURE 18.1.154 - Pes Planus

IV. Pes Cavus
   A. High-arched foot; high longitudinal plantar arch of foot
   B. Mostly idiopathic; can be associated with neurological and muscular disorders or Charcot-Marie-Tooth disease
   C. Imbalance between strong plantar flexion and weak dorsiflexion
   D. Diagnosis
      1. Mainly clinical
      2. X-ray of foot and ankle joint
   E. Management
      1. Corrective shoes and physiotherapy
      2. Surgery in case of resistant pes cavus

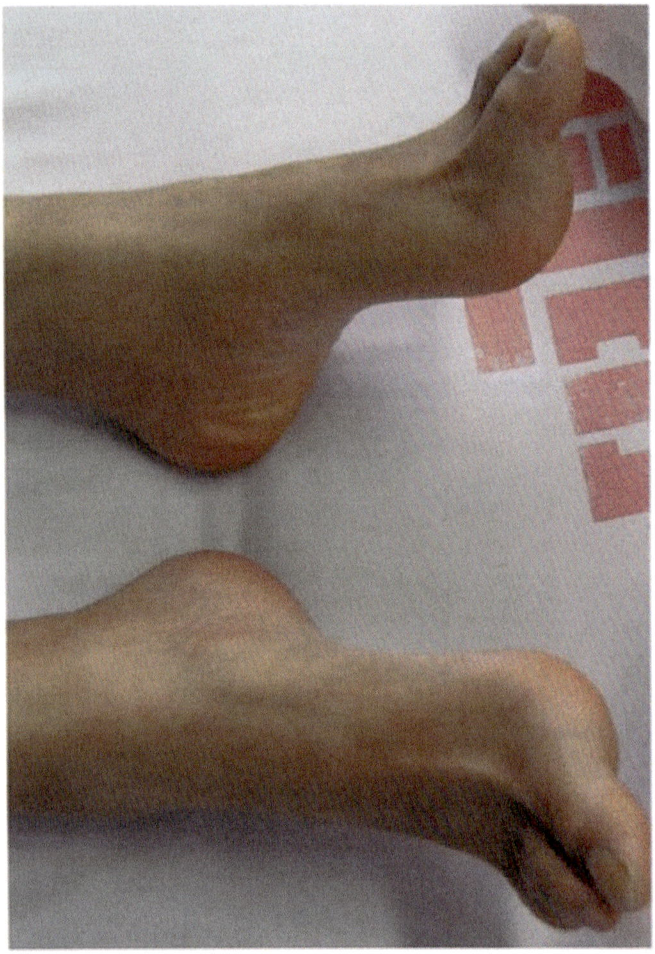

FIGURE 18.1.155 - Pes Cavus

REVIEW QUESTIONS

1. A 3-month-old boy is brought to his primary care physician by his parents because of a deformed foot. Physical examination shows adduction of the forefoot with convex lateral border and concave medial border. The hindfoot is in a neutral position. What is the most likely prognosis of this patient's condition?

   - **The most likely prognosis of this patient's condition is spontaneous resolution.**
   - This 3-month-old boy presents with a deformed foot.
   - Physical examination shows adduction of the forefoot with convex lateral border and concave medial border. The hindfoot is in a neutral position.
   - This is a classic description of metatarsus adductus.
   - Metatarsus adductus resolves spontaneously most of the time. Corrective shoes or casts may be needed for resistant cases.

2. A 6-month-old baby girl is brought to her primary care physician because of a deformity in both of her feet. Physical examination shows the posterior tibial muscles of the child is larger compared to the other muscles. X-ray of the child's feet shows, the long axes of the talus and calcaneus bones are parallel. Based on this child's diagnosis which additional feature would be expected on physical examination of the child's feet?

   A. Normal plantar flexion
   B. Toes turned outwards
   C. High arch
   D. Heel turned outwards

   - **The correct answer is option C.**
   - This 6-month-old baby girl presents with a deformity of both feet.
   - Physical examination is notable for dominance of posterior tibial muscles.
   - On X-ray of the feet, talocalcaneal parallelism is noted.
   - Based on these features, this child most likely has a club foot deformity.
   - The mnemonic CAVE can remember the features of club foot. This stands for Cavus of midfoot, which causes a high arch; Adductus of forefoot, where toes are turned inwards; Varus of hindfoot, where the heel turns inwards; and Equinus of hindfoot, which is abnormal plantar flexion.
   - Options A, B, and D are all incorrect because they represent the opposite of what would be expected in a club foot deformity.

Pediatrics | Section 37: MSK Disorders: Orthopedic Injuries

I. Clavicular Fracture
   A. Most common birth trauma
   B. Commonly seen in children and adolescents with fall on the shoulder
   C. Most common fracture site: junction of lateral and middle segments
   D. Clinical features
      1. Sagging of shoulder, short clavicle, skin tenting
      2. Symptoms of neurovascular involvement (e.g. weak pulses in upper extremity, brachial plexus injury)
   E. Diagnosis
      1. Physical examination shows swelling and concomitant injuries
      2. X-ray is best initial test; ultrasound in neonates
      3. CT/MRI if there is neurovascular involvement
   F. Management
      1. Midshaft fracture: conservative treatment with shoulder sling; surgery is reserved for largely displaced fractures
      2. Lateral segment fracture: shoulder sling; consider surgical plating or pinning for unstable fracture
      3. Medial segment fracture: shoulder sling

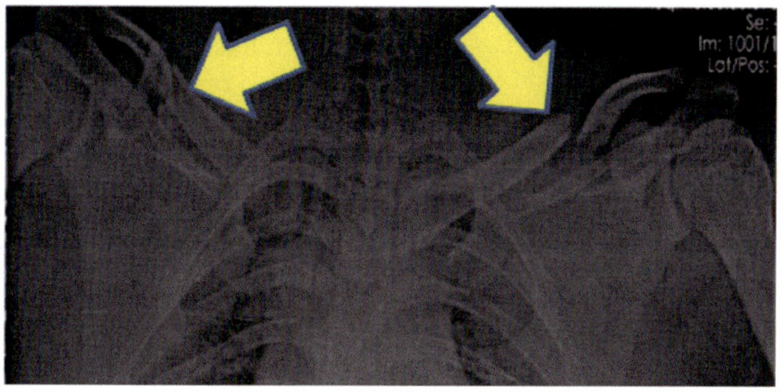

FIGURE 18.1.156 - Chest X-ray: Clavicular Fracture

II. Greenstick Fracture
      a. Partial thickness fracture
   A. Cortex and periosteum of the tension side (convex) are interrupted but these of compression side (concave) remain intact
   B. Angulation might be present
   C. Mostly present in diaphysis of radius, ulna, and fibula
   D. Most commonly due to fall on an outstretched hand
   E. Other risk factors: vitamin D deficiency, malnutrition
   F. Clinical features: pain on palpation, decreased range of motion of affected extremity
   G. Diagnosis: X-ray shows fracture line that doesn't travel throughout the bone
   H. Treatment
      1. Immobilization with cast
      2. Closed reduction is considered if there is excessive angulation

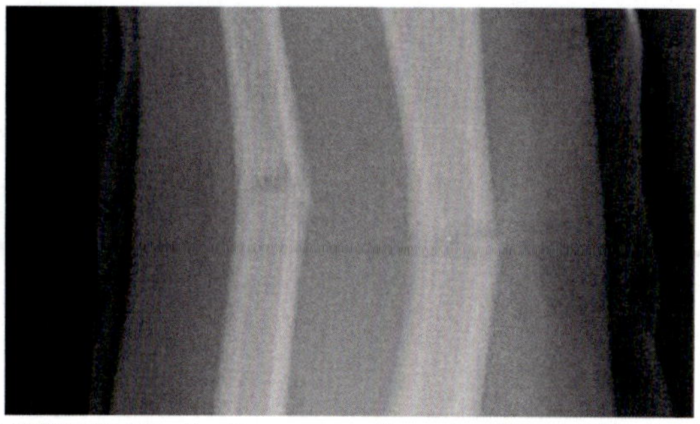

FIGURE 18.1.157 - X-ray of Arm: Greenstick Fracture

III. Torus Fracture
   A. Buckle fracture
   B. Cortex and periosteum are interrupted at the compression side (concave surface), whereas these of tension side are intact
   C. Mostly no angulation
   D. Most common site: distal radius at metadiaphyseal junction
   E. Diagnosis: X-ray
   F. Treatment: immobilization with cast for few weeks

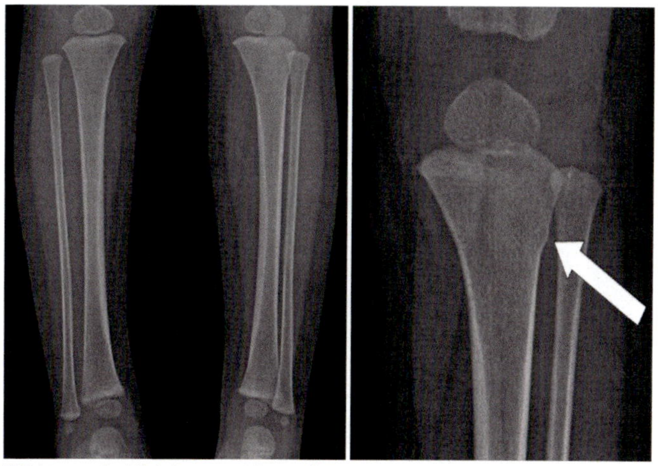

FIGURE 18.1.158 - X-ray of Tibia: Torus Fracture

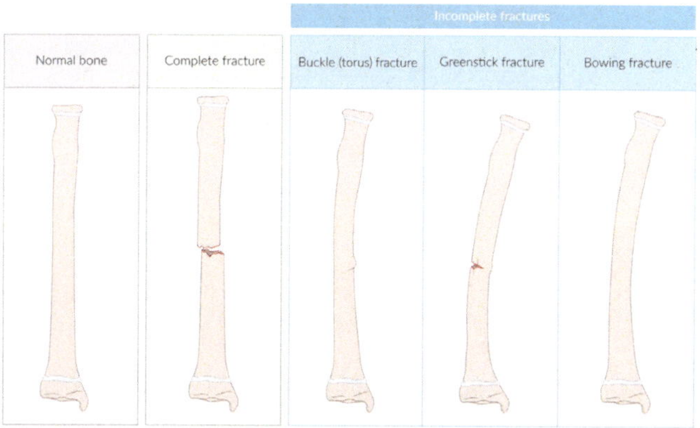

FIGURE 18.1.159 - Torus Fracture vs. Greenstick Fracture

IV. Nursemaid's Elbow
   A. Radial head subluxation in the presence of immature annular ligament
   B. Axial traction of radius during elbow extension (e.g. child is pulled up quickly or swinged)
   C. Mostly seen in children < 5 years of age
   D. Clinical findings
      1. Arm held flexed and pronated
      2. Pain with movement but no swelling
   E. Diagnosis
      1. Clinical diagnosis; X-ray is not required
   F. Treatment
      1. Closed reduction maneuvers: therapeutic and diagnostic
      2. Hyperpronation of forearm while applying pressure on radial head
      3. Supination of forearm and flexion of elbow while applying pressure on radial head

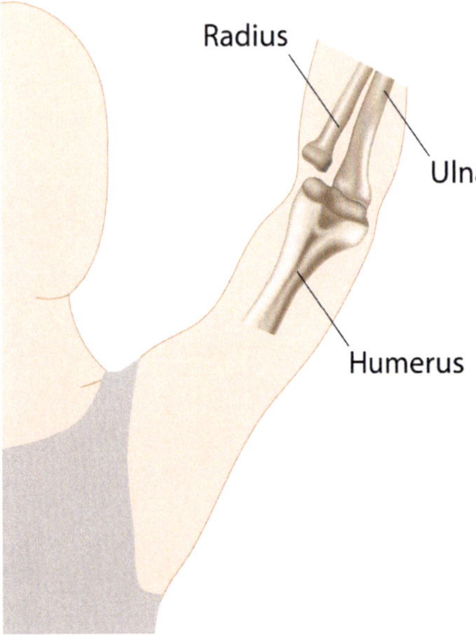

FIGURE 18.1.160 - Nursemaid's Elbow

V. Osgood-Schlatter Disease
   A. Tibial tuberosity apophysitis due to overuse of quadriceps muscle
   B. Mostly seen in adolescents (9 - 14 years)
   C. Excessive running and jumping during the adolescence causes microtrauma to the tibial tuberosity, leading to traction apophysitis
   D. Clinical findings
      1. Anterior knee pain which aggravates with activity and is reproduced with leg extension against resistance
   E. Diagnosis
      1. X-ray: soft tissue swelling, fragmented tubercle, elevated tubercle
   F. Treatment
      1. Conservative management with rest, ice, and NSAIDs
      2. Quadriceps strengthening and stretching exercises

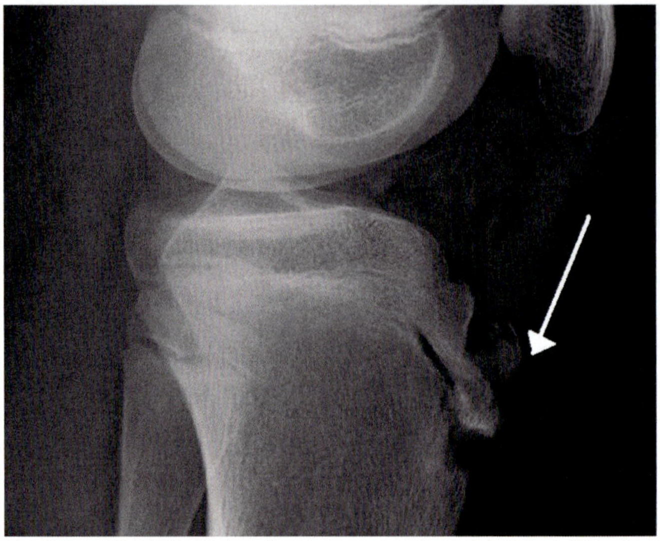

FIGURE 18.1.161 - X-ray of Knee Joint: Osgood-Schlatter Disease

VI. Salter-Harris Fracture
   A. Growth plate fracture
   B. During the time of growth spurts when puberty begins
   C. Most common sites: distal radius and distal humerus
   D. Clinical findings
      1. Joint pain, focal tenderness, swelling, decreased range of motion, inability to bear weight
   E. Diagnosis
      1. X-ray shows widening of the physis; MRI if X-ray is inconclusive
   F. Treatment
      1. Type I and II: closed reduction with cast immobilization; consider surgery if severe
      2. Type III and IV: ORIF (open reduction and internal fixation)
      3. Type V: usually diagnosed late so varies according to age
   G. Complications
      1. Growth arrest due to growth plate involvement
      2. Limb length discrepancies

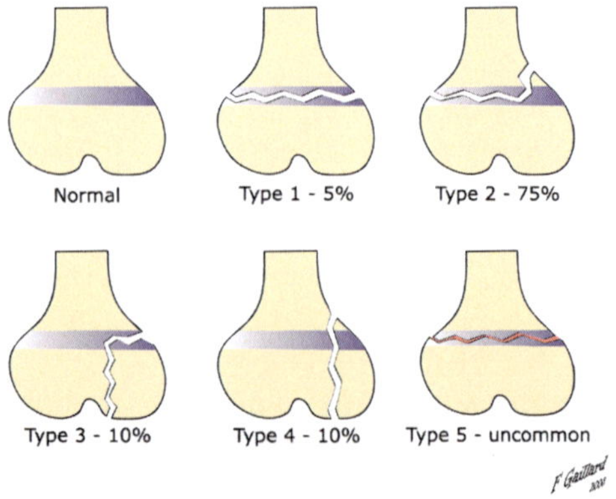

FIGURE 18.1.162 - Types of Salter-Harris Fracture

REVIEW QUESTIONS

1. A 3-year-old girl is brought to the emergency department due to right-sided hand pain after falling on an outstretched hand while she was playing. The physical examination shows distal radial tenderness on the right side. Wrist X-ray in AP view shows a partial thickness fracture at the tension site with an intact compression site. How can this patient's condition be distinguished from torus fracture?

    - **This patient's condition, a greenstick fracture, is characterized by a disrupted tension side and an intact compression side. In contrast, torus fracture is characterized by a disrupted compression side and an intact tension side.**
    - This patient presents with right-sided hand pain after falling on an outstretched hand.
    - The physical examination shows distal radial tenderness.
    - X-ray reveals a partial thickness fracture at the tension site with an intact compression site.
    - This is a classic description of greenstick fracture.

2. A 15-year-old boy is accompanied to the clinic by his father due to a painful right knee. He is a football player and his knee pain has interfered with his practice sessions. The physical examination shows swelling and tenderness below patella without warmth or erythema. Knee X-ray in lateral view shows elevation of right tibial tubercle. In addition to conservative measures, which type of exercise will likely alleviate this patient's symptoms?

    - **Quadriceps stretching and strengthening exercises will likely alleviate this patient's symptoms.**
    - This 15-year-old boy reports a painful right knee.
    - The physical examination shows swelling and tenderness below patella without warmth or erythema.
    - Leg X-ray shows elevation of right tibial tubercle.
    - These clues suggest the diagnosis of Osgood-Schlatter disease.
    - In addition to conversative measures like ice, NSAIDs, and rest, patients with Osgood-Schlatter disease benefit from quadriceps stretching and strengthening exercises.

3. A 6-year-old girl is brought to the emergency department due to left-sided hand pain after falling on an outstretched hand at school. Her vital signs are within normal limits. The physical examination shows a patient in severe distress along with left-sided distal radial tenderness. Wrist X-ray in AP view shows transverse lucency across the radial metaphysis, growth plate, and epiphysis. Which type of Salter-Harris fracture does this patient most likely have?

    A. Type I
    B. Type II
    C. Type III
    D. Type IV
    E. Type V

    - **The correct answer is option D.**
    - This 6-year-old girl presents with left-sided hand pain after falling on an outstretched hand at school.
    - The physical examination shows a patient in severe distress along with left-sided distal radial tenderness.
    - X-ray reveals a transverse lucency across the radial metaphysis, growth plate, and epiphysis. These X-ray findings are classic for type IV Salter-Harris fracture.
    - Type IV fracture is the only one involving all three parts - metaphysis, growth plate, and epiphysis.
    - Option A is incorrect because type I Salter-Harris fracture is characterized by a transverse fracture across the growth plate.
    - Option B is incorrect because type II fracture involves metaphysis and the growth plate.
    - Option C is incorrect because type III fracture involves epiphysis and the growth plate.
    - Option E is incorrect because type V Salter-Harris fracture is characterized by a crush injury of the growth plate.

Pediatrics | Section 38: Bilious Vomiting

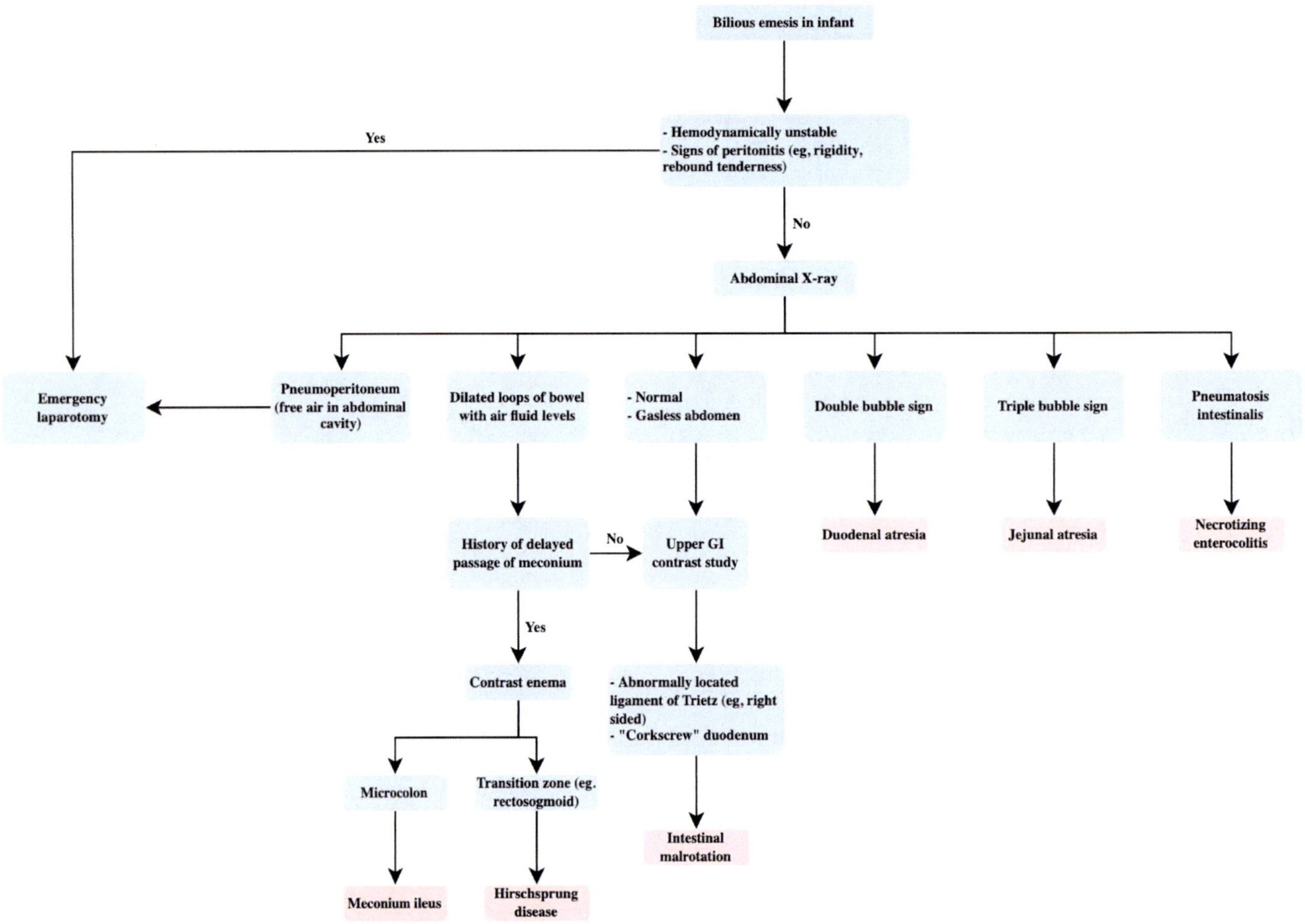

FIGURE 18.1.163 - Algorithm for Bilious Vomiting

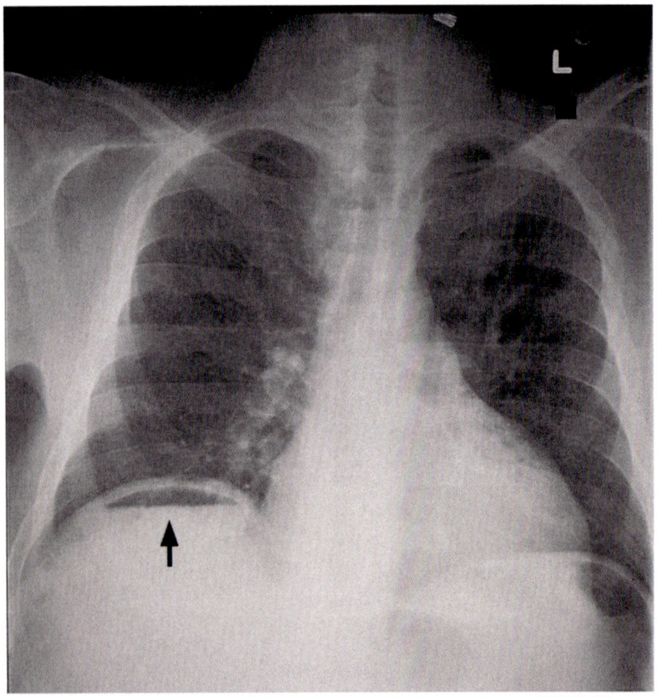

FIGURE 18.1.164 - Chest X-Ray Showing Pneumoperitoneum

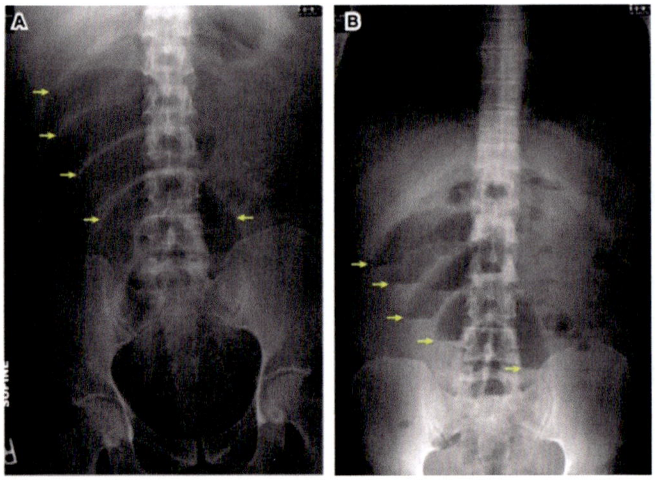

FIGURE 18.1.165 - Abdominal X-Ray Showing Dilated Loops of Bowel (Left) and Air-Fluid Levels (Right)

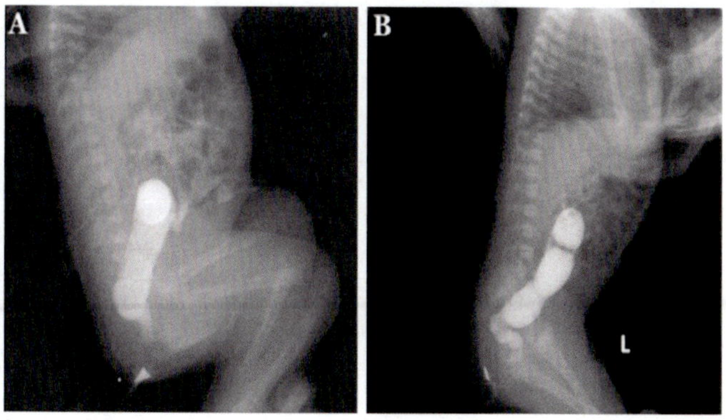

"Accuracy of transition zone in contrast enema to predict intraoperative aganglionosis level in patients with Hirschsprung disease" by Zikrul Haikal et al., BMC Research Notes is licensed under CC BY 4.0; Cropped by Physeo

FIGURE 18.1.166 - X-Ray with Contrast Enema Showing the Transition Zone in Hirschsprung's Disease

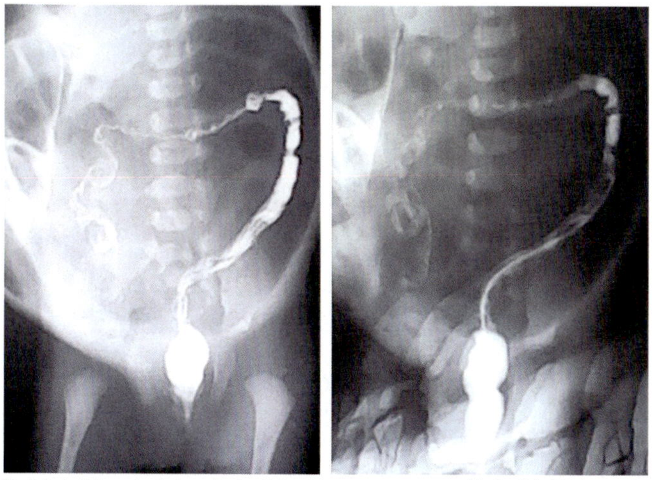

"Radiological diagnosis of microcolon in a 5-day old neonate: a case report" by Danfulani Mohammed et al., World Journal of Advanced Research and Reviews is licensed under CC BY 4.0

FIGURE 18.1.167- X-Ray with Contrast Enema Showing a Microcolon

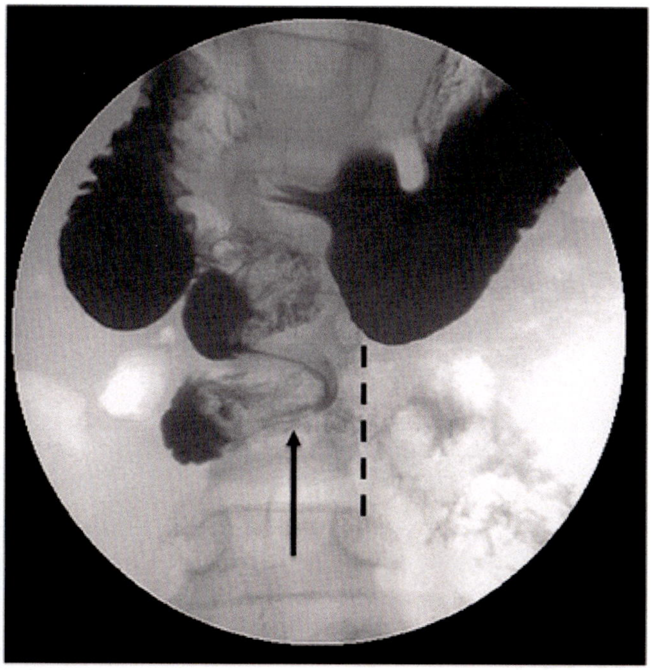

"Intestinal malrotation as a misdiagnosis of pediatric colchicine resistant familial Mediterranean fever" by Merav Heshin-Bekenstein and Philip J. Hashkes, Pediatric Rheumatology is licensed under CC BY 4.0

FIGURE 18.1.168 - X-Ray with Contrast Showing the Corkscrew Sign

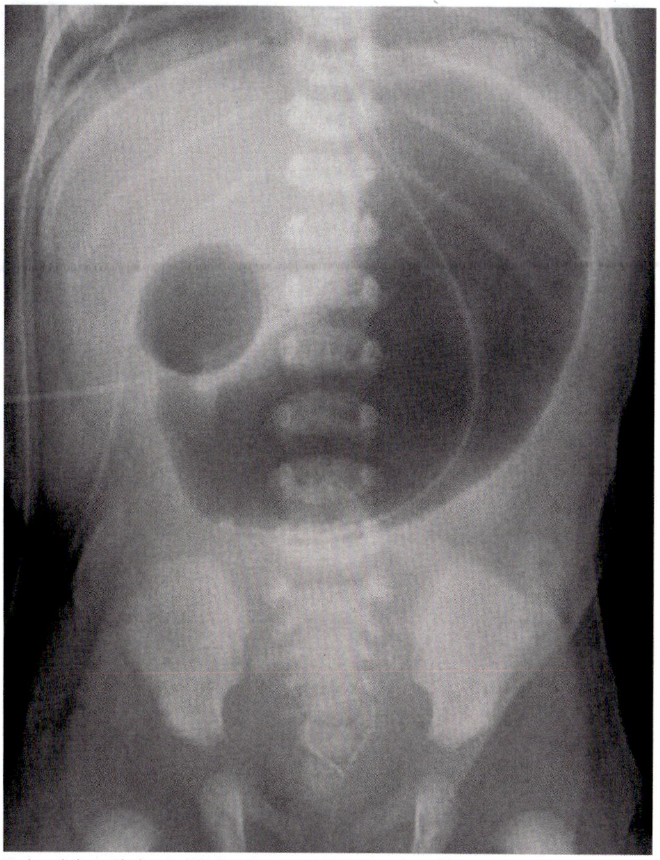

Kinderradiologie Olgahospital Klinikum Stuttgart, CC BY-SA 3.0 <https://creativecommons.org/licenses/by-sa/3.0>, via Wikimedia Commons

FIGURE 18.1.169 - Abdominal X-Ray Showing the Double-Bubble Sign

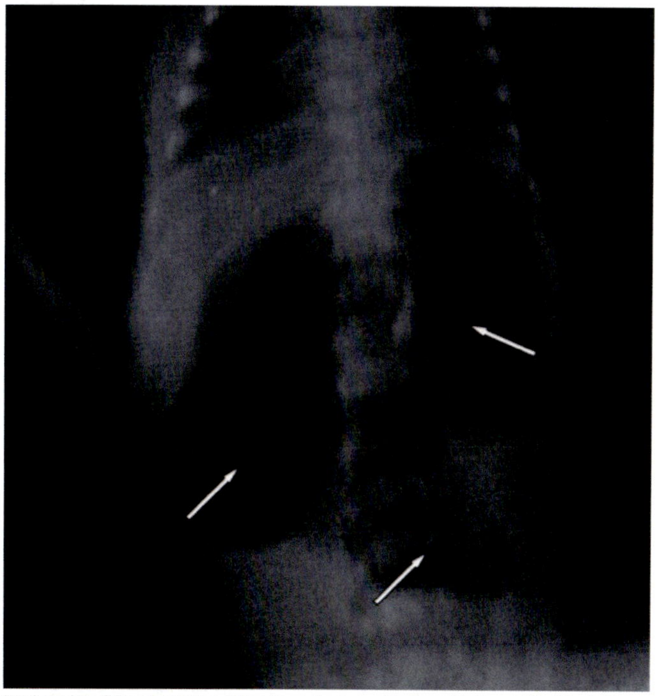

"Apple Peel Small Bowel, A Review of Four Cases: Surgical and Radiographic Aspects" by Akinola RA, Osuoji RI, Journal of Nepal Pediatric Society is licensed under CC BY 4.0

FIGURE 18.1.170 - Abdominal X-Ray Showing the Triple-Bubble Sign

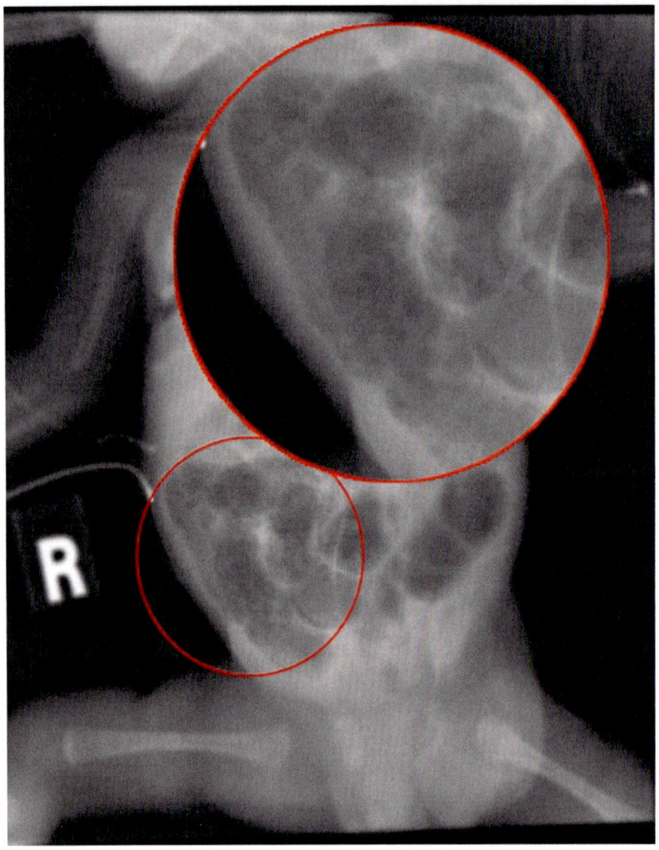

FIGURE 18.1.171 - Abdominal X-Ray of a Patient with Necrotizing Enterocolitis

REVIEW QUESTIONS

1. A 4-week-old baby boy is brought to the emergency department by his parents because of bilious vomiting and bloody stools for the past 5 hours. He was born at 32 weeks of gestation via emergency C-section due to maternal HELLP syndrome. His birth weight was 1 kg (2.5 kg - 4 kg) and length was 40 cm (46 cm - 56 cm). Vital signs show a temperature of 40° C (104° F), blood pressure of 60/40 mmHg, heart rate of 167 beats/min, and respiratory rate of 66 breaths/min. Physical examination shows abdominal distension and rigidity. Which of the following is the best next step in the management?

    A. Abdominal CT scan
    B. Upper GI contrast study
    C. Contrast enema
    D. Emergency laparotomy

- **The correct answer is option D.**
- This infant presents with vomiting and bloody stools for the past 5 hours.
- He was born prematurely at 32 weeks of gestation due to maternal HELLP syndrome.
- He had a very low birth weight of 1 kg and a shorter-than-normal length of 40 cm.
- Vital signs show a high fever of 40° C, hypotension with blood pressure of 60/40 mmHg, tachycardia with a heart rate of 167 beats/min, and tachypnea with a respiratory rate of 66 breaths/min.
- Physical examination shows abdominal distension and rigidity concerning for peritonitis.
- Considering his prematurity and very low birth weight, along with his other symptoms, there is high suspicion for necrotizing enterocolitis.
- The best next step in the management of an unstable infant with signs of peritonitis and bilious vomiting is an emergency laparotomy.
- Options A, B, and C are incorrect because abdominal CT scan, upper GI contrast study, and contrast enema are time-consuming and would not add any diagnostic value to this patient's emergent condition.

TABLES & FIGURES

TABLE 18.1.1 - Developmental Milestones from 2 Months to 12 Months....9
TABLE 18.1.2 - Developmental Milestones from 1.5 Years to 5 Years....9
TABLE 18.1.3 - Homocystinuria and Marfan Syndrome Characteristics....24
TABLE 18.1.4 - APGAR Score....25
TABLE 18.1.5 - Extracranial Injuries....26
TABLE 18.1.6 - Neonatal Jaundice....29
TABLE 18.1.7 - Neonatal Respiratory Pathologies....31
TABLE 18.1.8 - Pediatric Gastrointestinal Diseases....34
TABLE 18.1.9 - Pediatric Gastrointestinal Diseases....38
TABLE 18.1.10 - Congenital B Cell Immunodeficiencies....47
TABLE 18.1.11 - DiGeorge Syndrome....51
TABLE 18.1.12 - Congenital T-Cell Immunodeficiencies....55
TABLE 18.1.13 - Severe Combined Immunodeficiency and Wiskott Aldrich Syndrome....59
TABLE 18.1.14 - Hyper-IgM Syndrome and Ataxia-Telangiectasia....63
TABLE 18.1.15 - Summary of Chronic Granulomatous Disease and Myeloperoxidase Deficiency....66
TABLE 18.1.16 - Congenital Phagocyte Defects....69
TABLE 18.1.17 - Juvenile Idiopathic Arthritis....75
TABLE 18.1.18 - Epiglottitis and Croup....81
TABLE 18.1.19 - Infections of the Respiratory Tract....85
TABLE 18.1.20 - Viral Exanthems....90
TABLE 18.1.21 - Common Screening Recommendations....91
TABLE 18.1.22 - Key Immunizations....92
TABLE 18.1.23 - Immunization Schedule....92
TABLE 18.1.24 - Vital Signs and Growth Measurements....94
TABLE 18.1.25 - Key Features of Pediatric Physical Examination....95
TABLE 18.1.26 - Normal vs. Abnormal Sexual Behaviors of Toddlers and School-Aged Children....100
FIGURE 18.1.1 - Raking Grasp....8
FIGURE 18.1.2 - Pincer Grasp....8
FIGURE 18.1.3 - Growth Chart....10
FIGURE 18.1.4 - Tanner Stages....12
FIGURE 18.1.5 - Unilateral Sharply Contoured Cafe-Au-Lait Spots....13
FIGURE 18.1.6 - X-ray: Central Hyperlucency....13
FIGURE 18.1.7 - Fundoscopy: "Cherry-Red" Spot on the Macula....18
FIGURE 18.1.8 - Light Microscopy: Foam Cells in Niemann-Pick Disease....18
FIGURE 18.1.9 - Angiokeratomas....18
FIGURE 18.1.10 - Light Microscopy: Globoid Cells in Krabbe Disease....20
FIGURE 18.1.11 - X-ray of the Hip: Avascular Necrosis of the Femur Head....20
FIGURE 18.1.12 - Light Microscopy: "Crumpled Tissue Paper" Macrophages in Gaucher Disease....20
FIGURE 18.1.13 - Corneal Clouding in Hurler Syndrome....21
FIGURE 18.1.14 - Infant with Bilateral Cataracts....22
FIGURE 18.1.15 - Pathways of Homocysteine Metabolism....22
FIGURE 18.1.16 - Marfanoid Habitus....23
FIGURE 18.1.17 - Homocystinuria....23
FIGURE 18.1.18 - Cystine Crystals in Urine....23
FIGURE 18.1.19 - Acrocyanosis....25
FIGURE 18.1.20 - Extracranial Injuries....25
FIGURE 18.1.21 - MRI of the Brain: Bilateral Hyperintensities in the Basal Ganglia (Kernicterus)....27
FIGURE 18.1.22 - Jaundice....27
FIGURE 18.1.23 - Bhutani Nomogram....28
FIGURE 18.1.24 - X-ray of the Chest: Reticulogranular "Ground-Glass" Densities and Air Bronchograms in Respiratory Distress Syndrome....30
FIGURE 18.1.25 - X-ray of the Chest: Asymmetric, Patchy Opacities in Meconium Aspiration Syndrome....30
FIGURE 18.1.26 - Hypertrophic Pyloric Stenosis....32
FIGURE 18.1.27 - Abdominal Ultrasound: Thickened Pyloric Walls and Narrowed Pyloric Channel in Hypertrophic Pyloric Stenosis....32

FIGURE 18.1.28 - Intussusception....32
FIGURE 18.1.29 - Light Microscopy: Peyer Patches....32
FIGURE 18.1.30 - Midgut Malrotation....33
FIGURE 18.1.31 - Barium Enema: Intestinal Malrotation....33
FIGURE 18.1.32 - X-ray of the Abdomen: "Coffee-Bean" Sign in Sigmoid Volvulus....33
FIGURE 18.1.33 - Meckel's Diverticulum....36
FIGURE 18.1.34 - Meckel Scan....36
FIGURE 18.1.35 - Hirschsprung Disease....37
FIGURE 18.1.36 - Abdominal X-ray: Pneumatosis Intestinalis in Necrotizing Enterocolitis....37
FIGURE 18.1.37 - Chest X-ray: Pneumoperitoneum....38
FIGURE 18.1.38 - Pathway of Normal Descent of the Testicle....40
FIGURE 18.1.39 - The Urinary System....40
FIGURE 18.1.41 - Management of Febrile UTI in Child < 2 Years of Age....41
FIGURE 18.1.42 - Voiding Cystourethrogram: Bilateral Vesicoureteral Reflux....41
FIGURE 18.1.43 - Voiding Cystourethrogram: Unilateral Vesicoureteral Reflux....41
FIGURE 18.1.44 - Potter Sequence....42
FIGURE 18.1.45 - Posterior Urethral Valve....42
FIGURE 18.1.46 - Bladder Exstrophy....44
FIGURE 18.1.47 - Epispadias....44
FIGURE 18.1.48 - Hypospadias....44
FIGURE 18.1.49 - Phimosis (Before Surgical Treatment)....45
FIGURE 18.1.50 - After Surgical Treatment of Phimosis....45
FIGURE 18.1.51 - The Uvula and Tonsils....46
FIGURE 18.1.52 - Steps of Antibody Production....46
FIGURE 18.1.53 - Pharyngeal Pouches, Clefts, and Arches....49
FIGURE 18.1.54 - The Pharyngeal Apparatus....49
FIGURE 18.1.55 - The Thymus....49
FIGURE 18.1.56 - Cleft Palate....49
FIGURE 18.1.57 - Hypertelorism....50
FIGURE 18.1.58 - Chest X-ray of a Healthy Infant....50
FIGURE 18.1.59 - Chest X-ray of a Healthy Adult....50
FIGURE 18.1.60 - Normal Heart....50
FIGURE 18.1.61 - Truncus Arteriosus....50
FIGURE 18.1.62 - Tetralogy of Fallot....50
FIGURE 18.1.63 - Chest X-ray: "Boot-Shaped" Heart in Tetralogy of Fallot....51
FIGURE 18.1.64 - Fluorescence In-Situ Hybridization: Normal Cells vs Cells with *22q11.2* Microdeletion....51
FIGURE 18.1.65 - Atopic Dermatitis....53
FIGURE 18.1.66 - A Cutaneous Abscess....53
FIGURE 18.1.67 - Scoliosis....53
FIGURE 18.1.68 - *Eczematous Dermatitis*....54
FIGURE 18.1.69 - Onychomycosis....54
FIGURE 18.1.70 - Patient with Oral Thrush Due to Infection with *Candida*....57, 60
FIGURE 18.1.71 - Chest X-ray Showing Bilateral "Ground-Glass"....57
FIGURE 18.1.72 - Healthy Baby Chest X-Ray....57
FIGURE 18.1.73 - Healthy Adult Chest X-Ray....58
FIGURE 18.1.74 - Eczema in Patient with Wiskott-Aldrich Syndrome....58
FIGURE 18.1.75 - Petechiae and Purpura in Patients with Thrombocytopenia....58
FIGURE 18.1.76 - Leukoplakia....60
FIGURE 18.1.77 - Class Switching of B Cells....62
FIGURE 18.1.78 - Ocular Telangiectasias....62
FIGURE 18.1.79 - Cutaneous Telangiectasias....63
FIGURE 18.1.80 - Pathophysiology of Chronic Granulomatous Disease....65, 68
FIGURE 18.1.81 - Dihydrorhodamine Test Results....65
FIGURE 18.1.82 - Phagocytes Under a Gram Stain....65
FIGURE 18.1.83 - Process of Leukocytes Traveling Within Blood Vessel to Site of Infection....68
FIGURE 18.1.84 - Blood Smear of a Patient with Chediak Higashi Syndrome....68
FIGURE 18.1.85 - Edema and Swelling in Hereditary Angioedema....71
FIGURE 18.1.86 - Edema and Swelling in Hereditary Angioedema....72
FIGURE 18.1.87 - Kinin System....72
FIGURE 18.1.88 - Petechiae and Purpura in Meningococcal Meningitis....72
FIGURE 18.1.89 - Different Types of Juvenile Idiopathic Arthritis....74

FIGURE 18.1.90 - Anterior Uveitis....74
FIGURE 18.1.91 - Child with Systemic Juvenile Idiopathic Arthritis....76
FIGURE 18.1.92 - Patient with Swollen Metatarsal & Interphalangeal Joints....76
FIGURE 18.1.93 - Salmon-Colored Rash....77
FIGURE 18.1.94 - Less Common Types of Juvenile Idiopathic Arthritis....77
FIGURE 18.1.95 - Tripod Positioning....79
FIGURE 18.1.96 - Laryngoscopy: "Cherry-Red" Epiglottis....79
FIGURE 18.1.97 - Lateral Neck X-ray of a Healthy Person....79
FIGURE 18.1.98 - Lateral Neck X-ray: "Thumbprint Sign" in Epiglottitis....80
FIGURE 18.1.99 - Chest X-ray: "Steeple Sign" in Croup....80
FIGURE 18.1.100 - Chest X-Ray: Hyperinflation and Areas of Atelectasis in Bronchiolitis....83
FIGURE 18.1.101 - Chest X-ray: Patchy Consolidation in Bacterial Pneumonia....84
FIGURE 18.1.102 - Chest X-ray: Bilateral, Diffuse Opacities in Viral Pneumonia....84
FIGURE 18.1.103 - Slapped-Cheek Rash of Erythema Infectiosum....88
FIGURE 18.1.104 - Koplik Spots....88
FIGURE 18.1.105 - Measles Exanthem....88
FIGURE 18.1.106 - Rubella Exanthem....89
FIGURE 18.1.107 - Roseola Exanthem....89
FIGURE 18.1.108 - Varicella Exanthem....89
FIGURE 18.1.109 - Intussusception....93
FIGURE 18.1.110 - Pediatric Growth Chart....94
FIGURE 18.1.111- Cranial Birth Injuries....95
FIGURE 18.1.112 - Strabismus....95
FIGURE 18.1.113 - Normal Red Reflex vs. Abnormal Red Reflex....96
FIGURE 18.1.114 - Abdominal X-ray: Pneumatosis Intestinalis....96
FIGURE 18.1.115 - X-ray: Congenital Diaphragmatic Hernia....96
FIGURE 18.1.116 - Irritant Diaper Dermatitis....96
FIGURE 18.1.117 - Candida Diaper Dermatitis....96
FIGURE 18.1.118 - Barlow & Ortolani Tests....96, 112
FIGURE 18.1.119 - Galeazzi Sign....97, 113
FIGURE 18.1.120 - Club Foot....97
FIGURE 18.1.121 - Metatarsus Adductus....97, 116
FIGURE 18.1.122 - "Rib-Humping" Sign in Scoliosis....97
FIGURE 18.1.123 - Congenital Dermal Melanocytosis....97
FIGURE 18.1.124 - Congenital Dermal Melanocytosis....99
FIGURE 18.1.125 - Cupping Bruises....99
FIGURE 18.1.126 - X-ray of the Humerus: Spiral Fracture....100
FIGURE 18.1.127 - Patient With Superior Vena Cava Syndrome....102
FIGURE 18.1.128 - Peripheral Blood Smear Showing Immature Lymphoblasts....102
FIGURE 18.1.129 - Biopsy Showing Homer-Wright Rosettes....104
FIGURE 18.1.130 - Clinical Features of Beckwith-Wiedemann Syndrome....104
FIGURE 18.1.131 - X-ray Knee Showing Codman Triangle and Sunburst Pattern in Osteosarcoma....106
FIGURE 18.1.132 - X-ray Knee Showing "Onion Skin" Periosteal Reaction in Ewing Sarcoma....106
FIGURE 18.1.133 - Biopsy Showing Anaplastic Blue Cells in Ewing Sarcoma....106
FIGURE 18.1.134 - Equinovarus Deformity....108
FIGURE 18.1.135 - Corticospinal Tract....108
FIGURE 18.1.136 - Spastic Cerebral Palsy....108
FIGURE 18.1.137 - MRI of the Brain: Cystic Periventricular Malacia....109
FIGURE 18.1.139 - CT Scan of the Head: Intracerebral Hemorrhage....109
FIGURE 18.1.140 - CT Scan of the Head: Intraventricular Hemorrhage....109
FIGURE 18.1.141 - Botulinum Toxin....109
FIGURE 18.1.142 - Subluxation and Displacement of Femoral Head After Necrosis....111
FIGURE 18.1.143 - Pelvic X-Ray Showing Flattening of Both Femoral Heads....111
FIGURE 18.1.144 - Pelvic X-Ray Showing Necrosis and Fragmentation of the left Femoral Head....111
FIGURE 18.1.145 - X-Ray of the Hip Joint....112
FIGURE 18.1.146 - X-Ray Showing Slipped Capital Femoral Epiphysis, Before and After Surgical Intervention....112
FIGURE 18.1.147 - Trendelenburg Gait....113
FIGURE 18.1.148 - Normal Hip Ultrasound in an Infant....113
FIGURE 18.1.149 - Pelvic X-Ray Showing Developmental Dysplasia of the Right Hip....114
FIGURE 18.1.150 - Baby Wearing Pavlik Harness....114
FIGURE 18.1.151 - Diagram of Baby Wearing a Pavlik Harness....114

FIGURE 18.1.152 - Hip Spica Cast Treatment....114
FIGURE 18.1.153 - Club Foot....116
FIGURE 18.1.154 - Pes Planus....116
FIGURE 18.1.155 - Pes Cavus....117
FIGURE 18.1.156 - Chest X-ray: Clavicular Fracture....118
FIGURE 18.1.157 - X-ray of Arm: Greenstick Fracture....118
FIGURE 18.1.158 - X-ray of Tibia: Torus Fracture....118
FIGURE 18.1.159 - Torus Fracture vs. Greenstick Fracture....118
FIGURE 18.1.160 - Nursemaid's Elbow....119
FIGURE 18.1.161 - X-ray of Knee Joint: Osgood-Schlatter Disease....119
FIGURE 18.1.162 - Types of Salter-Harris Fracture....119
FIGURE 18.1.163 - Algorithm for Bilious Vomiting....121
FIGURE 18.1.164 - Chest X-Ray Showing Pneumoperitoneum....121
FIGURE 18.1.165 - Abdominal X-Ray Showing Dilated Loops of Bowel (Left) and Air-Fluid Levels (Right)....121
FIGURE 18.1.166 - X-Ray with Contrast Enema Showing the Transition Zone in Hirschsprung's Disease....122
FIGURE 18.1.167- X-Ray with Contrast Enema Showing a Microcolon....122
FIGURE 18.1.168 - X-Ray with Contrast Showing the Corkscrew Sign....122
FIGURE 18.1.169 - Abdominal X-Ray Showing the Double-Bubble Sign....122
FIGURE 18.1.170 - Abdominal X-Ray Showing the Triple-Bubble Sign....122
FIGURE 18.1.171 - Abdominal X-Ray of a Patient with Necrotizing Enterocolitis....123

Made in United States
Orlando, FL
04 November 2026

90201390R00076